Advance in Gluten-Free Diet

Advance in Gluten-Free Diet

Editor

Paolo Usai-Satta

MDPI • Basel • Beijing • Wuhan • Barcelona • Belgrade • Manchester • Tokyo • Cluj • Tianjin

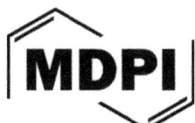

Editor
Paolo Usai-Satta
Brotzu Hospital, Piazzale Alessandro Ricchi
Cagliari, Italy

Editorial Office
MDPI
St. Alban-Anlage 66
4052 Basel, Switzerland

This is a reprint of articles from the Special Issue published online in the open access journal *Nutrients* (ISSN 2072-6643) (available at: https://www.mdpi.com/journal/nutrients/special_issues/gluten).

For citation purposes, cite each article independently as indicated on the article page online and as indicated below:

LastName, A.A.; LastName, B.B.; LastName, C.C. Article Title. *Journal Name* **Year**, *Volume Number*, Page Range.

ISBN 978-3-03943-871-6 (Hbk)
ISBN 978-3-03943-872-3 (PDF)

© 2020 by the authors. Articles in this book are Open Access and distributed under the Creative Commons Attribution (CC BY) license, which allows users to download, copy and build upon published articles, as long as the author and publisher are properly credited, which ensures maximum dissemination and a wider impact of our publications.

The book as a whole is distributed by MDPI under the terms and conditions of the Creative Commons license CC BY-NC-ND.

Contents

About the Editor vii

Paolo Usai-Satta and Mariantonia Lai
New Perspectives on Gluten-Free Diet
Reprinted from: *Nutrients* **2020**, *12*, 3540, doi:10.3390/nu12113540 1

Aureliusz Kosendiak, Piotr Stanikowski, Dorota Domagała and Waldemar Gustaw
Gluten-Free Diet in Prisons in Poland: Nutrient Contents and Implementation of Dietary Reference Intake Standards
Reprinted from: *Nutrients* **2020**, *12*, 2829, doi:10.3390/nu12092829 5

Violeta Fajardo, María Purificación González, María Martínez, María de Lourdes Samaniego-Vaesken, María Achón, Natalia Úbeda and Elena Alonso-Aperte
Updated Food Composition Database for Cereal-Based Gluten Free Products in Spain: Is Reformulation Moving on?
Reprinted from: *Nutrients* **2020**, *12*, 2369, doi:10.3390/nu12082369 17

Raffaele Borghini, Natascia De Amicis, Antonino Bella, Nicoletta Greco, Giuseppe Donato and Antonio Picarelli
Beneficial Effects of a Low-Nickel Diet on Relapsing IBS-Like and Extraintestinal Symptoms of Celiac Patients during a Proper Gluten-Free Diet: Nickel Allergic Contact Mucositis in Suspected Non-Responsive Celiac Disease
Reprinted from: *Nutrients* **2020**, *12*, 2277, doi:10.3390/nu12082277 35

Alice Scricciolo, Luca Elli, Luisa Doneda, Karla A Bascunan, Federica Branchi, Francesca Ferretti, Maurizio Vecchi and Leda Roncoroni
Efficacy of a High-Iron Dietary Intervention in Women with Celiac Disease and Iron Deficiency without Anemia: A Clinical Trial
Reprinted from: *Nutrients* **2020**, *12*, 2122, doi:10.3390/nu12072122 49

Michael D. E. Potter, Kerith Duncanson, Michael P. Jones, Marjorie M. Walker, Simon Keely and Nicholas J. Talley
Wheat Sensitivity and Functional Dyspepsia: A Pilot, Double-Blind, Randomized, Placebo-Controlled Dietary Crossover Trial with Novel Challenge Protocol
Reprinted from: *Nutrients* **2020**, *12*, 1947, doi:10.3390/nu12071947 57

Antonio Carroccio, Pasquale Mansueto, Maurizio Soresi, Francesca Fayer, Diana Di Liberto, Erika Monguzzi, Marianna Lo Pizzo, Francesco La Blasca, Girolamo Geraci, Alice Pecoraro, Francesco Dieli and Detlef Schuppan
Wheat Consumption Leads to Immune Activation and Symptom Worsening in Patients with Familial Mediterranean Fever: A Pilot Randomized Trial
Reprinted from: *Nutrients* **2020**, *12*, 1127, doi:10.3390/nu12041127 67

Paolo Usai-Satta, Gabrio Bassotti, Massimo Bellini, Francesco Oppia, Mariantonia Lai and Francesco Cabras
Irritable Bowel Syndrome and Gluten-Related Disorders
Reprinted from: *Nutrients* **2020**, *12*, 1117, doi:10.3390/nu12041117 79

Massimo Bellini, Sara Tonarelli, Maria Gloria Mumolo, Francesco Bronzini, Andrea Pancetti, Lorenzo Bertani, Francesco Costa, Angelo Ricchiuti, Nicola de Bortoli, Santino Marchi and Alessandra Rossi
Low Fermentable Oligo- Di- and Mono-Saccharides and Polyols (FODMAPs) or Gluten Free Diet: What Is Best for Irritable Bowel Syndrome?
Reprinted from: *Nutrients* **2020**, *12*, 3368, doi:10.3390/nu12113368 . . . . **87**

About the Editor

Paolo Usai-Satta (MD) is a gastroenterologist with expertise in celiac disease, alimentary intolerance, and digestive pathophysiology. He is a clinical physician at the Gastroenterology Unit of Brotzu hospital in Cagliari (Italy). His research is focused on Irritable bowel syndrome, alimentary intolerances, celiac disease, and digestive motility disorders. He is a member of the European Society of NeuroGastroenterology and Motility and the Italian Group of Digestive Motility. He is also advisor board member and general secretary of the Italian Association of Hospital Gastroenterology (AIGO).

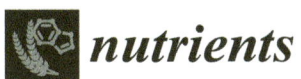

Editorial

New Perspectives on Gluten-Free Diet

Paolo Usai-Satta [1],* and Mariantonia Lai [2]

1. Gastroenterology Unit, Brotzu Hospital, 09124 Cagliari, Italy
2. Gastroenterology Unit, University of Cagliari, 09042 Monserrato, Italy; laimariantonia@gmail.com
* Correspondence: paolousai@aob.it; Tel.: +39-070-539-395

Received: 9 November 2020; Accepted: 17 November 2020; Published: 18 November 2020

Celiac disease (CD) is a permanent, chronic, gluten-sensitive disorder characterized by small intestinal inflammation and malabsorption in genetically predisposed individuals [1]. In addition, a self-reported gluten/wheat sensitivity without the diagnostic features of CD has recently been named non-celiac gluten/wheat sensitivity (NCGWS) [2].

The only effective and safe treatment for CD and gluten-related disorders (GRD) is a lifelong, strict exclusion of gluten, the so-called gluten-free diet (GFD). In this respect, there are new concepts and perspectives regarding GFD and its impact on clinical practice.

This Special Issue, entitled "Advance in Gluten-Free Diet", comprises eight peer-reviewed papers reporting on different points of view regarding GFD in different clinical conditions.

In detail, the interplay between irritable bowel syndrome (IBS) and GRD, the role of GFD compared to low fermentable oligo/di/monosaccharides and polyols (FODMAP) diet (LFD) in IBS and functional dyspepsia (FD), the role of a low nickel diet in CD on GFD with persistent IBS-like symptoms, the efficacy of high-iron diet in CD with iron deficiency without anemia, the current reformulation of gluten-free food composition in Spain, the nutritional value of GFD in Polish CD prisoners and the symptoms worsening after wheat ingestion in familial Mediterranean fever are discussed in this Special Issue.

IBS is frequently associated with CD, and IBS symptoms may also overlap and be similar to those associated with NCGWS. In addition, many patients with CD have persistent digestive symptoms despite a strict GFD. This can be due to a higher frequency of IBS in CD patients compared to the general population. On the other hand, many different dietary approaches have been recently suggested for IBS and a GFD is considered a therapeutic option in a subset of IBS patients [3].

In their review, Bellini et al. [4] discuss the evidence regarding two of the most advised diets for IBS, the GFD and the LFD. A GFD is less restrictive and easer to follow than LFD. On the other hand, according to recent evidence, LFD is the most effective dietary intervention suggested for treating IBS, and it is included in the most updated guidelines. Unfortunately, the clinical trials regarding the dietary intervention for IBS are of low quality. The problem is the difficulty in setting up randomized double-blind controlled trials which objectively evaluate clinical results without the risk of a nocebo/placebo effect.

Similarly to IBS, both GFD and LFD could improve symptoms in patients with FD. In a double-blind, randomized, placebo controlled pilot trial, Potter et al. [5] have evaluated the role of this diet (specifically gluten and fructan) in patients with FD. A combined GFD–LFD led to an overall improvement in dyspeptic symptoms but this result was not significant. Otherwise, a specific food trigger was not identified. The authors consequently suggest further larger studies to confirm these data.

As hypothesized by Borghini et al. [6], a nickel-rich diet could exacerbate or relapse IBS-like symptoms in CD patients on strict GFD. In fact, many gluten-free foods are high in nickel content. In their study, 20 celiac patients on GFD, with persistent digestive symptoms and with positive patch test for nickel-mucositis, consumed a low-nickel diet. The result was an overall improvement in digestive symptoms in CD patients, with significant effects for 10 out of 24 symptoms (according to

Gastrointestinal Symptom Rating Scale modified questionnaire). The impact of a nickel-rich diet on CD could be a clinical and scientific challenge for further studies to address.

Iron deficiency without anemia is a common clinical scenario in CD despite a strict GFD. A recommended approach to this condition is not yet defined. Scricciolo et al. [7] have compared a 12-week iron-rich diet to iron supplementation with ferrous sulfate in 22 celiac adult women. At the end of the treatments, both well tolerated, ferritin levels were statistically higher in the ferrous sulfate group. An iron-rich diet can be, however, recommended in patients who do not tolerate pharmacological supplementation.

The objective of the paper by Fajardo et al. [8] was to develop a nutritional food composition database including cereal-based gluten-free products available in Spain. A comprehensive database of 629 products was achieved. Gluten-free products were primarily composed of rice and/or corn flour. The most common added fat was sunflower oil, followed by palm fat, olive oil and cocoa. Xanthan gum was the most frequently employed fiber. Nutritional deficiencies have been described for CD patients on GFD and an updated quality assessment of available products is needed for further improvement in gluten-free product development.

A special clinical setting for CD patients can be represented by the prison population. The risk of nutritional deficiencies may be a real problem for CD prisoners due to the limited possibilities of external quality control. In the study by Kosendiak et al. [9], the nutritional value of GFD and regular diet meals served in 10 Polish prisons were assessed. GFD was characterized by lower average energy content in 11 out 14 essential nutrients. Greater quality control of GFD meals served in catering facilities should be recommended.

Finally, Carroccio et al. [10] have identified a clinical association between self-reported NCGWS and familial Mediterranean fever (FMF). In their pilot randomized trial, the authors have evaluated clinical and innate immune responses to wheat (compared to rice) challenge. In six NCGWS/FMF female patients, wheat ingestion exacerbated clinical and immunological features of FMF. These findings may suggest new clinical scenarios in the management of FMF.

In conclusion, the different perspectives presented in this Special Issue confirm that the gluten-free diet is currently a clinically and scientifically challenging topic. We would like to thank all the authors and the editorial team of *Nutrients* for their precious contributions.

Funding: This review received no external funding.

Conflicts of Interest: The authors declare no conflict of interest.

References

1. Kelly, C.P.; Bai, J.C.; Liu, E.; Leffler, D.A. Advances in diagnosis and management of celiac disease. *Gastroenterology* **2015**, *148*, 1175–1186. [CrossRef] [PubMed]
2. Catassi, C.; Alaedini, A.; Bojarski, C.; Bonaz, B.; Bouma, G.; Carroccio, A.; Castillejo, G.; De Magistris, L.; Dieterich, W.; Di Liberto, D.; et al. The Overlapping Area of Non-Celiac Gluten Sensitivity (NCGS) and Wheat-Sensitive Irritable Bowel Syndrome (IBS): An Update. *Nutrients* **2017**, *9*, 1268. [CrossRef] [PubMed]
3. Usai Satta, P.; Bassotti, G.; Bellini, M.; Oppia, F.; Lai, M.; Cabras, F. Irritable bowel syndrome and gluten-related disorders. *Nutrients* **2020**, *12*, 1117. [CrossRef] [PubMed]
4. Bellini, M.; Tonarelli, S.; Mumolo, M.G.; Bronzini, F.; Pancetti, A.; Bertani, L.; Costa, F.; Ricchiuti, A.; de Bortoli, N.; Marchi, S.; et al. Low Fermentable Oligo- Di- and Mono-Saccharides and Polyols (FODMAPs) or Gluten Free Diet: What Is Best for Irritable Bowel Syndrome? *Nutrients* **2020**, *12*, 3368. [CrossRef] [PubMed]
5. Potter, M.D.E.; Duncanson, K.; Jones, M.P.; Walker, M.M.; Keely, S.; Talley, N.J. Wheat Sensitivity and Functional Dyspepsia: A Pilot, Double-Blind, Randomized, Placebo-Controlled Dietary Crossover Trial with Novel Challenge Protocol. *Nutrients* **2020**, *12*, 1947. [CrossRef] [PubMed]

6. Borghini, R.; De Amicis, N.; Bella, A.; Greco, N.; Donato, G.; Picarelli, A. Beneficial Effects of a Low-Nickel Diet on Relapsing IBS-Like and Extraintestinal Symptoms of Celiac Patients during a Proper Gluten-Free Diet: Nickel Allergic Contact Mucositis in Suspected Non-Responsive Celiac Disease. *Nutrients* **2020**, *12*, 2277. [CrossRef] [PubMed]
7. Scricciolo, A.; Elli, L.; Doneda, L.; Bascunan, K.A.; Branchi, F.; Ferretti, F.; Vecchi, M.; Roncoroni, L. Efficacy of a High-Iron Dietary Intervention in Women with Celiac Disease and Iron Deficiency without Anemia: A Clinical Trial. *Nutrients* **2020**, *12*, 2122. [CrossRef] [PubMed]
8. Fajardo, V.; González, M.P.; Martínez, M.; Samaniego-Vaesken, M.L.; Achón, M.; Úbeda, N.; Alonso-Aperte, E. Updated Food Composition Database for Cereal-Based Gluten Free Products in Spain: Is Reformulation Moving on? *Nutrients* **2020**, *12*, 2369. [CrossRef] [PubMed]
9. Kosendiak, A.; Stanikowski, P.; Domagała, D.; Gustaw, W. Gluten-Free Diet in Prisons in Poland: Nutrient Contents and Implementation of Dietary Reference Intake Standards. *Nutrients* **2020**, *12*, 2829. [CrossRef] [PubMed]
10. Carroccio, A.; Mansueto, P.; Soresi, M.; Fayer, F.; Di Liberto, D.; Monguzzi, E.; Lo Pizzo, M.; La Blasca, F.; Geraci, G.; Pecoraro, A.; et al. Wheat Consumption Leads to Immune Activation and Symptom Worsening in Patients with Familial Mediterranean Fever: A Pilot Randomized Trial. *Nutrients* **2020**, *12*, 1127. [CrossRef] [PubMed]

Publisher's Note: MDPI stays neutral with regard to jurisdictional claims in published maps and institutional affiliations.

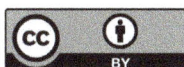

© 2020 by the authors. Licensee MDPI, Basel, Switzerland. This article is an open access article distributed under the terms and conditions of the Creative Commons Attribution (CC BY) license (http://creativecommons.org/licenses/by/4.0/).

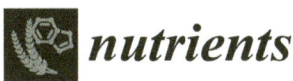 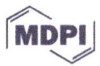

Article

Gluten-Free Diet in Prisons in Poland: Nutrient Contents and Implementation of Dietary Reference Intake Standards

Aureliusz Kosendiak [1], Piotr Stanikowski [2,*], Dorota Domagała [3] and Waldemar Gustaw [2]

[1] Study of Physical Education and Sport, Wroclaw Medical University, 51-601 Wroclaw, Poland; aureliusz.kosendiak@umed.wroc.pl
[2] Department of Plant Food Technology and Gastronomy, Faculty of Food Science and Biotechnology, University of Life Sciences in Lublin, 20-704 Lublin, Poland; waldemar.gustaw@up.lublin.pl
[3] Department of Applied Mathematics and Computer Science, Faculty of Production Engineering, University of Life Sciences in Lublin, 20-612 Lublin, Poland; dorota.domagala@up.lublin.pl
* Correspondence: piotr.stanikowski@up.lublin.pl; Tel.: +48-81-462-33-09

Received: 15 August 2020; Accepted: 12 September 2020; Published: 16 September 2020

Abstract: The gluten-free diet (GFD) requires special attention from nutritionists due to the potential risk of nutrient deficiencies in its users. This risk may be greater when this type of nutrition is implemented in prisons due to the limited possibilities of external control, a low catering budget for meals, and insufficiently defined recommendations regulating nutrition for prisoners. The aim of the present study was to assess the nutritional value of GFD and regular diet meals served in some Polish prisons and to compare the values to the dietary reference intake (DRI) standards. Using a specialized computer program, 7-day menus of both types of diet provided in 10 prisons were analyzed. The percentage coverage of the DRI was calculated based on the recommendations of the Polish National Food and Nutrition Institute. GFD was characterized by lower average contents of energy and 11 out of 14 essential nutrients, i.e., protein, carbohydrates, dietary fiber, starch, ash, sodium, calcium, iron, zinc, folate, and vitamin B_{12}. The average content of phosphorus, niacin, and riboflavin in the gluten-free diet was higher than that in the regular diet. It was shown that the meals in GFD and the regular diet did not provide the recommended amounts of calcium (38 and 44% DRI, respectively), vitamin D (29 and 30% DRI), vitamin C (86 and 76% DRI), and folate (51 and 56% DRI). In turn, the supply of sodium, phosphorus, copper, and vitamins A and B_6 substantially exceeded the recommended levels. The results indicate a need for greater quality control of GFD meals served in catering facilities. It is also necessary to develop legal provisions that will regulate more specifically the nutrition for prisoners in terms of an adequate supply of minerals and vitamins.

Keywords: gluten-free diet; celiac disease; dietary reference intake; prison diets

1. Introduction

Gluten is a general term given to the following fractions of protein: gliadins, glutenins, hordein, and secalin. These protein fractions are found in four grains, i.e., wheat, rye, barley, and triticale. Oats are inherently gluten-free but may be contaminated with wheat during growing or processing [1]. The ingestion of gluten can trigger an array of conditions; they are designated by a broader term "gluten-related disorders". They are divided into disorders with autoimmune pathogenesis, including celiac disease (CD), disorders characterized by allergic mechanisms, which include wheat allergy, and the controversial non-celiac gluten sensitivity, whose causes are neither autoimmune nor allergic in nature [2].

CD is a common chronic immune-mediated small bowel enteropathy resulting from gluten exposure in genetically susceptible individuals [3]. It is generally acknowledged that about 1% of the general population have CD [4]. In the US population, a higher proportion of persons living at latitudes of 35° North or greater have CD or avoid gluten than persons living south of this latitude, independent of the race or ethnicity, socioeconomic status, or body mass index [5]. Unfortunately, there are no data about the prevalence rate of CD and other gluten-related disorders in the health statistics reports on prisoners [6–8].

Currently, the only effective treatment available for CD is a strict life-long gluten-free diet (GFD), since it leads to resolution of intestinal and extraintestinal symptoms, negativity of autoantibodies, and regrowth of intestinal villi. In addition, the diet exerts a partial protective effect on several complications. However, these crucial advantages are accompanied by some disadvantages, including a negative impact on the quality of life, psychological problems, fear of involuntary/inadvertent gluten contamination, increased cardiovascular risk, and frequent severe constipation [9]. Gluten-free food products are substantially more expensive than regular equivalents. Replacement of commonly consumed cereal staple foods in GFDs with gluten-free equivalents may be associated with an increased supply of fat, saturated fatty acids, salt, and sugar [10]. GFD may lead to possible nutrient deficiencies of fiber [11,12], folate [11–14], vitamin D [11,14,15], calcium [11,12,14,16], magnesium [11,12,16], iron [12,14], zinc [16], selenium [16], and iodine [14]. To increase the supply of nutrients, it is recommended to include legume and pseudo-cereal products (especially amaranth, quinoa, and soybeans) in GFD. They are a better source of fat, fiber, high-quality protein, and minerals than the frequently served corn and rice [17].

The aim of the present study was to assess the nutritional value of gluten-free and regular diet meals served in some Polish prisons and to compare the values to the dietary reference intake standards.

2. Materials and Methods

2.1. General Information

The study was approved by the Director-General of the Prison Service in Poland on 3 December 2018. Next, a request for access to the menus was sent in an electronic or paper form to all the institutions. In total, 88 prisons responded to the request. Ten independent prisons, all serving gluten-free diet, were selected for the investigations, i.e., detention centers in Gdańsk, Poznań, Suwałki, and Wrocław and prisons in Dębica, Grądy Woniecko, Iława, Nysa, Strzelce Opolskie (No. 2), and Włodawa. Most of the institutions were male prisons, whereas three facilities were female and male prisons. All prisons were designed for adults.

2.2. Analysis of Energy and Nutrient Content

The analysis involved 7-day GFD menus (from different seasons) and 7-day regular diet menus (from different seasons) provided by each prison in 2018. The regular diet was served to all healthy adult prisoners, while the GFD was prescribed by medical staff [18]. In the study, 140 all-day menus consisting of breakfast, lunch, and supper were analyzed. A typical GFD breakfast usually consisted of puffed rice cakes, margarine, sandwich meats, jam, and an apple/vegetable. Various types of soup and a dish composed of meat, potatoes/white rice, and side salad were served for lunch. Supper mostly included white rice/puffed rice cakes, margarine, and sandwich meats/cottage cheese. With each meal, prisoners made tea themselves. The calculations did not include food that prisoners were able to buy at least three times a month in the prison canteen or food parcels that prisoners received once a month from their relatives [19].

The quantitative analysis was carried out with the use of specialized software DietetykPro (DietetykPro, Wrocław, Poland), which mainly incorporates Polish Food Composition databases developed at the National Food and Nutrition Institute in Warsaw [20] and the database of the United States Department of Agriculture [21]. All food products specified in the menus and inventory reports were analyzed. The inventory reports included names of the food products and their quantity in kilograms/liters used in the kitchen to prepare all meals. Ready meals included in the software database were not taken into account in the analysis. The study involved assessment of 31 parameters of daily food rations: energy value, total protein, total fat, total carbohydrate, dietary fiber, sucrose, starch, cholesterol, fatty acids (saturated, monounsaturated, polyunsaturated), ash, minerals (sodium, potassium, calcium, phosphorus, magnesium, iron, zinc, copper), and vitamins A (as retinol activity equivalents), retinol, B_1, B_2, niacin, B_6, B_{12}, C, D, E, and folate (as dietary folate equivalents). The results took into account averaged technological losses caused by heat treatment: folate and vitamin C, 50%; vitamin B_1, 30%; vitamin B_6, 25%; vitamins A, E, retinol, and niacin, 20%; and other parameters, 10%. Next, the percentage of the dietary reference intake (DRI) was calculated based on nutrition standards for the Polish population [22]. Since approximately 57% of male prisoners in Poland in 2019 were in the age range of 31–50 [8], the calculations were based on recommendations for this group. For calculation of energy requirement, the physical activity level (PAL) of 1.4 was adopted.

Next, the DietetykPro and Microsoft Excel software was used to analyze the consumption of food groups. The classification of the food groups and subgroups was based on the Polish Food Composition databases [20]. Certain modifications in the classification have been introduced for better presentation of the differences between the analyzed diets. In the "cereal products" group, a sub-group "puffed rice cakes" has been added. The "vegetables and vegetable products" group has been supplemented with a "starchy roots" sub-group, and the "legumes" sub-group has been removed and analyzed as a separate "legumes" group.

2.3. Statistical Analysis

The statistical analysis was carried out using the Microsoft Excel 2020 and Statistica 13.1 program (StatSoft, Cracow, Poland). Welch's test was used to check whether the type of diet had an effect on the average content of the analyzed nutrients, energy, and daily consumption of the food groups. In the next step, 95% confidence intervals for differences between the means of 15 components significantly differing between the gluten-free and regular diets were determined. Similarly, such intervals were calculated for the daily consumption of seven food groups which were differed significantly in both types of diet.

3. Results

3.1. Energy and Macronutrients

The daily energy supply met the recommendations of the Polish National Food and Nutrition Institute in the case of GFD, but exceeded the recommended values by 108 kcal in the regular diet (Table 1). The supply of saturated fatty acids (SFA) was 24.5 g in the case of GFD and 26.3 g in the case of the regular diet, which exceeded the recommended values. SFAs covered approx. 9.0% of total energy intake.

Table 1. Energy and macronutrients provided in prisons (n = 10) menus per person per day and the age-specific dietary reference intake (DRI).

Observed Component	Recommended	Gluten-Free Diet Mean ± SD	Regular Diet Mean ± SD
Energy (kcal)	2100–2600 (EER)	2405.5 ± 355.6	2708.0 ± 258.6
Protein (g)	50–77 (RDA)	82.3 ± 10.5	90.6 ± 15.6
Fat (g)	70–87 [1]	72.4 ± 21.2	79.0 ± 18.2
SFA (g)	max. 17.6–21.1	24.5 ± 11.9	26.3 ± 8.9
MUFA (g)	N.A.	28.6 ± 9.1	31.0 ± 7.3
PUFA (g)	N.A.	15.4 ± 6.5	16.2 ± 5.3
Cholesterol (mg)	N.A.	244.0 ± 128.6	243.7 ± 106.4
Carbohydrates (g)	130 (RDA)	370.7 ± 57.6	429.5 ± 40.9
Starch (g)	N.A.	149.4 ± 48.0	293.4 ± 37.4
Sucrose (g)	N.A.	53.7 ± 18.1	52.5 ± 18.6
Fiber (g)	25 (AI)	30.0 ± 6.4	37.3 ± 6.4

[1] 30% of energy from fats; EER estimated energy requirement; RDA recommended dietary allowance; SFA saturated fatty acids; MUFA monounsaturated fatty acids; PUFA polyunsaturated fatty acids; AI adequate intake; N.A. not available.

3.2. Micronutrients

The average supply of micronutrients in the daily food ration is presented in Table 2. In comparison with the recommendations, excess consumption of three minerals, i.e., sodium, phosphorus, and copper, was recorded in both diets. A particularly high supply was recorded in the case of sodium. The consumption of potassium slightly exceeded the recommended values. The supply of magnesium, iron, and zinc was close to the reference values. The lowest supply of all minerals was recorded for calcium. Its intake in GFD was 378.7 mg, which covered 38% of DRI. The intake of this element in the regular diet was 440.3 mg, which represented 44% of DRI.

Table 2. Micronutrients provided in prisons ($n = 10$) menus per person per day and the age-specific dietary reference intake (DRI).

Observed Component	Recommended	Gluten-Free Diet		Regular Diet	
		Mean ± SD	% of DRI	Mean ± SD	% of DRI
Ash (g)	N.A.	18.2 ± 3.6	N.A.	29.7 ± 4.3	N.A.
Sodium (mg)	1500 (AI)	3073.9 ± 910.8	205	7727.0 ± 1569.7	515
Potassium (mg)	3500 (AI)	4892.6 ± 1143.5	140	4628.8 ± 1049.5	132
Calcium (mg)	1000 (RDA)	378.7 ± 163.2	38	440.3 ± 128.5	44
Phosphorus (mg)	700 (RDA)	1452.0 ± 172.8	207	1377.6 ± 218.3	197
Magnesium (mg)	420 (RDA)	410.3 ± 76.2	98	397.4 ± 76.4	95
Iron (mg)	10 (RDA)	11.6 ± 2.7	116	16.1 ± 4.4	161
Zinc (mg)	11 (RDA)	12.2 ± 2.4	111	13.4 ± 2.3	122
Copper (mg)	0.9 (RDA)	1.7 ± 0.3	189	1.8 ± 0.4	200
Vitamin A (µg)	900 (RDA)	2776.3 ± 1319.0	308	2339.3 ± 2437.9	260
Retinol (µg)	N.A.	279.7 ± 211.2	N.A.	681.0 ± 2161.3	N.A.
Vitamin D (µg)	15 (AI)	4.3 ± 3.3	29	4.5 ± 4.3	30
Vitamin E (mg)	10 (AI)	12.0 ± 3.9	120	11.3 ± 3.5	113
Vitamin B_1 (mg)	1.3 (RDA)	1.4 ± 0.4	108	1.5 ± 0.4	115
Vitamin B_2 (mg)	1.3 (RDA)	1.3 ± 0.4	100	1.1 ± 0.7	85
Niacin (mg)	16 (RDA)	22.3 ± 4.9	139	19.7 ± 5.0	123
Vitamin B_6 (mg)	1.3 (RDA)	2.9 ± 0.5	223	3.0 ± 1.8	231
Vitamin B_{12} (µg)	2.4 (RDA)	2.1 ± 1.1	88	4.3 ± 5.5	179
Vitamin C (mg)	90 (RDA)	77.4 ± 33.9	86	68.1 ± 26.9	76
Folate (mg)	400 (RDA)	204.2 ± 52.2	51	222.2 ± 47.5	56

AI adequate intake; RDA recommended dietary allowance; N.A. not available.

The content of vitamins A and B_6 in the analyzed menus substantially exceeded the recommended values. In turn, the supply of vitamin D in both diets was very low, i.e., 4.3 and 4.5 µg, respectively. This only covered 29% of the recommended values in GFD and 30% in the regular diet. Both diets were characterized by a low intake of folate, covering approximately half of the DRI value.

3.3. Analysis of the Menus by Types of Diet

The gluten-free and regular diets differed statistically significantly in the content of energy and 14 nutrients: protein, carbohydrates, dietary fiber, starch, ash, sodium, calcium, phosphorus, iron, zinc, riboflavin, niacin, folate, and vitamin B_{12}. For the differences between the mean levels of the essential ingredients in the regular diet and GFD, 95% confidence intervals were determined (Table 3). GFD was characterized by lower average contents of energy and 11 of the 14 essential nutrients, i.e., protein, carbohydrates, dietary fiber, starch, ash, sodium, calcium, iron, zinc, folate, and vitamin B_{12}. The average content of phosphorus, niacin, and riboflavin in GFD was higher than in the regular diet.

Table 3. Lower and upper endpoints of a 95% confidence interval for the difference between mean regular and gluten-free diet.

Observed Component	$\bar{x}_r - \bar{x}_{gf}$	Lower Endpoint	Upper Endpoint
Energy (kcal)	302.49	198.58	406.40
Protein (g)	8.29	3.84	12.74
Carbohydrates (g)	58.78	42.09	75.47
Fiber (g)	7.34	5.21	9.47
Starch (g)	143.95	129.56	158.34
Ash (g)	11.48	10.15	12.82
Sodium (mg)	4653.14	4224.23	5082.04
Calcium (mg)	61.66	12.57	110.75
Phosphorus (mg)	−74.40	−140.21	−8.59
Iron (mg)	4.48	3.26	5.71
Zinc (mg)	1.28	0.48	2.08
Riboflavin (mg)	−0.23	−0.41	−0.05
Niacin (mg)	−2.59	−4.24	−0.95
Folate (mg)	18.06	1.39	34.73
Vitamin B$_{12}$ (µg)	2.21	0.89	3.52

$\bar{x}_r$—mean value for regular diet, $\bar{x}_{gf}$—mean value for gluten-free diet.

3.4. Analysis of the Food Group Consumption

In both types of diet, no consumption of products from the groups and subgroups "frozen fruits", "fruit, dried", "nuts", "seeds", and "beverages" was recorded (Table 4). Products from the subgroup "mushrooms" were served in only three prisons. In GFD, no products from the subgroups "pasta" (including gluten-free pasta), "breads and rolls" (including gluten-free breads and rolls) were served, and "legumes" were noted in only one object. The regular diet was characterized by no consumption of products from the subgroup "puffed rice cakes".

Table 4. Distribution of food group and sub-group consumption (g/day).

Food Groups and Sub-Groups	Gluten-Free Diet		Regular Diet	
	Mean	SD	Mean	SD
Cereal products	221.34	58.40	465.00	34.42
Grains, flours and starches	14.30	23.06	13.30	3.80
Groats	100.07	73.40	37.02	9.88
Pasta	0.00	0.00	22.89	9.45
Breads and rolls	0.00	0.00	391.17	30.66
Breakfast cereals	1.52	2.87	0.98	1.91
Puffed rice cakes	105.45	16.96	0.00	0.00
Vegetables and vegetable products	919.39	153.68	850.51	106.96
Vegetables, raw and boiled	402.27	91.11	326.52	68.22
Frozen vegetables	27.64	28.62	10.62	12.24
Vegetable products	3.75	4.56	77.70	44.63
Mushrooms	1.18	3.33	3.23	6.27
Starchy roots	484.55	104.96	432.45	77.71
Legumes	1.79	5.05	19.72	6.86
Fruits and fruit products	346.72	285.06	88.79	66.81
Fruit, raw	344.77	251.32	62.70	62.09
Frozen fruits	0.00	0.00	0.00	0.00
Fruit, dried	0.00	0.00	0.00	0.00
Fruit products	54.64	40.09	26.09	14.10
Nuts	0.00	0.00	0.00	0.00
Seeds	0.00	0.00	0.00	0.00

Table 4. Cont.

Food Groups and Sub-Groups	Gluten-Free Diet		Regular Diet	
	Mean	SD	Mean	SD
Milk and milk products	61.96	39.05	56.14	27.77
Meat and meat products	241.52	49.64	222.92	40.74
Fish, fish products and seafood	10.71	12.27	38.32	15.69
Eggs	15.73	22.94	10.86	7.27
Fats and oils	64.25	26.26	46.31	14.31
Sugar and confectionery	25.43	18.49	32.18	10.65
Beverages	0.00	0.00	0.00	0.00
Other products	14.52	9.10	38.12	9.86

Food groups are bolded in the table.

The regular diet and GFD differed significantly in terms of the consumption of products from the following food groups and subgroups: "cereal products", "groats", "vegetable products", "fish, fish products, and seafood", "fruits and fruit products", "fruit, raw", and "other products" (Table 5). In GFD, the consumption of products from the groups "groats", "fruits and fruit products", and "fruit, raw" was significantly higher than in the regular diet and significantly lower in the case of the other groups ("cereal products", "vegetable products", "fish, fish products and seafood", and "other products") than in the regular diet (Table 5).

Table 5. Lower and upper endpoints of a 95% confidence interval for the difference between mean regular and gluten-free diet.

Food Groups and Sub-Groups	$\bar{x}_R - \bar{x}_{GF}$	Lower Endpoint	Upper Endpoint
Cereal products	243.66	191.10	296.21
Groats	−63.05	−124.53	−1.57
Vegetable products	73.95	36.59	111.30
Fish, fish products and seafood	27.61	12.42	42.79
Fruits and fruit products	−257.93	−497.89	−17.96
Fruit, raw	−282.07	−493.83	−70.31
Other products	23.60	13.42	33.78

$\bar{x}_R$—mean value for regular diet, $\bar{x}_{GF}$—mean value for gluten-free diet.

4. Discussion

The investigations conducted by our team revealed inadequate quality of meals served in the Polish prisons. Compared to the regular diet, GFD was characterized by a significantly lower average level of energy and 11 nutrients: protein, carbohydrates, dietary fiber, starch, ash, sodium, calcium, iron, zinc, folate, and vitamin B_{12}. The mean content of phosphorus, niacin, and riboflavin was higher in GFD than in the regular diet.

The implementation of GFD involves exclusion of many food products. Wheat or mixed bread was found to be the basic food served for breakfast and supper in almost all diets available in the Polish prisons. It was mainly replaced with puffed rice cakes in the GFD meals. Therefore, the cost of GFD breakfast and supper was high, since puffed rice cakes were up to 10 times more expensive than bread, as shown by the inventory reports. Hence, prison meal planners tended to limit the amount of these products served for breakfast and supper even twice in comparison with the ration of bread served in these meals in the other diets. The difference in the consumption of cereal products between the regular diet and GFD, i.e., 243.66 g, probably had an impact on the supply of energy, protein, and carbohydrates, which was significantly higher in the regular diet. As suggested by Soto et al. [23], the difference in the energy value between GFD and regular diet meals may also be associated with the exclusion of breaded fried foods. Bread, rolls, and bread products contribute substantially to the supply of many nutrients. In the average Polish diet, these products provide 48.6% of manganese, 36.3% of carbohydrates, 35.4% of fiber, 24.9% of iron, 22.1% of copper, 21.1% of zinc, 21% of magnesium, and 20.7% of folate [24]. Therefore, the exclusion of bread from GFD may have resulted in the considerably lower consumption of such nutrients as fiber, iron, zinc, and folate, in comparison with the regular diet.

The average energy value was 2405.5 kcal/day in the GFD menus and 2708.0 kcal/day in the regular diet. The energy value in the latter diet was higher than the nutritional standards recommended for the Polish population (2100–2600 kcal) [22]. As specified by the regulations on nutrition for prisoners in Poland, meals should provide at least 2600 kcal [18]. In our opinion, these recommendations require personalization, which is supported by the varied physical activity [25] and excessive body weight in Polish prisoners [26].

The analysis of the menus did not show any disturbing observations regarding the supply of macronutrients in the diet. Only the consumption of SFAs exceeded the recommended values in both analyzed diets. However, no significantly higher consumption of this ingredient was detected in GFD, which is usually observed in patients with celiac disease [27]. This may be related to the higher SFA content in GF products than in their counterparts [28]. The lower supply of fiber in GFD compared to the regular diet indicated by the present results is in agreement with values reported by other authors [16,28,29]. The consumption of dietary fiber in GFD covered DRI, although it was significantly lower than in the regular diet. This may be related to the significantly higher consumption of groats, fruit, and fruit products in this diet compared to GFD, which we showed in the analysis of the consumption of the food groups. It is recommended that GFD meals should be enriched with fiber and minerals through consumption of legumes and pseudocereals [17]. The analysis conducted in the study showed very low consumption of legumes, which in the case of GFD were included in the menu in only one prison, whereas no pseudocereals were served. The main ingredient of lunch was white rice, while brown rice, which provides more fiber and many other health-beneficial food components [30], was not served at all. The analyzed GFD diets did not include oat, which is nutritious and a good source of fiber and can be safely consumed by patients with CD [31]. However, according to the recommendations of the Polish Association of People with Celiac Disease and the Gluten-Free Diet, oats and oat products in Poland are highly contaminated with gluten and therefore should not be used in the GFD [32].

To our knowledge, the large difference in the supply of sodium between the two analyzed diets was associated with the fact that the meal planners followed invalid provisions regulating the issue of nutrition in prisons in Poland [33]. These regulations recommended that the daily salt intake in therapeutic diets should be limited to 6 g per day. The analysis of the menus and inventory reports demonstrated that the regular diet and GFD were planned to contain 3 to 11 g and 0 to 3 g of table salt per day, respectively. We reported high levels of salt additions to prison meals in our previous investigations as well [34]. Besides the lower addition of salt to the dishes, the sodium content in GFD may also have been influenced by the exclusion of bread from the diet. Bread is a source of 17.5% of sodium in the average diet of the Polish population [24] and 23% of sodium in the diet of Polish hypertension patients [35]. As far as other minerals are concerned, a significantly low calcium intake was noted in both diets. The low calcium supply is reflected in the level of consumption of the respective food groups. The average consumption of milk and dairy products, which are the most important source of this mineral, was only 61.96 g in GFD and 56.14 g in the regular diet. An adequate supply of this mineral is particularly important in CD patients, due to the malabsorption of the nutrient, which may lead to development of bone diseases [36]. Individuals with undiagnosed and untreated CD are at the highest risk of malabsorption [37]. GFD was characterized by a significantly lower supply of calcium than the regular diet. There are inconsistent data showing differences in the supply of this component between GFD and regular diets. The results reported by Dall'Asta et al. [27] confirm our observations, whereas Wild et al. [16] suggest that patients with GFD may consume higher amounts of calcium than those with a non-GFD diet. There are also considerable differences in the supply of this nutrient to CD patients depending on their sex and age [38]. Due to the high supply of phosphorus, the menus analyzed in the present study had a very unfavorable Ca:P ratio, i.e., 0.26:1 in GFD and 0.32:1 in the regular diet. The correct ratio of these two minerals is 1.5:1 [39].

The supply of vitamins in both diets was especially high in the case of vitamins A and B_6. The consumption of vitamins C, vitamin D, and folate did not meet the recommended intake. An inadequate supply of these nutrients was also observed in other studies on the nutrition of Polish prisoners [34,40,41]. The high supply of vitamin A in the analyzed menus was probably related to the frequent use of margarine (30–90 g per day), which is obligatorily fortified with this vitamin in Poland. The large standard deviations in the case of the vitamin A supply were probably associated with the presence of fried pork liver in many menus for the convicts. The supply of vitamin B_6 in both diets covered over 200% of DRI. It is generally lower in the Polish population, as 16% of males and 36% of females do not consume or supplement its recommended amounts [42]. Vitamin D, the consumption of which in the daily food ration did not cover even half of the recommended amount, is especially important for celiac disease patients. It plays a key role in the regulation of immune response and may have an impact on CD [43]. As shown by research conducted in the USA, only 31% of prisoners have normal levels of this component in blood [44]. The cutaneous synthesis of this vitamin in prisoners may be lower than in the general population due to the limited time spent outdoors. However, deficiencies of this component have even been detected in 90% of individuals imprisoned in places with high sun exposure [45]. In our opinion, the low supply of vitamin C was probably caused by the limitation of the assortment of vegetables to a few cheapest ones, which are not a good source of this vitamin (beetroot, carrots, onions, and potatoes). Similarly, the range of fruit served in the diets sporadically was limited to apples. The infrequent presence of vegetables in the diets probably contributed to the low supply of folate. A significantly lower supply of this nutrient was noted in GFD, which may have been associated with the exclusion of many cereal products from this diet.

Analyses of the present results should take into account that the quality of GFD meals served in prisons may be influenced by the low catering budget allowance. This was evidenced by the results of our previous investigations of the nutrition for Polish prisoners, which demonstrated that the limited financial means resulted in a large reduction in the range of fruit and vegetables served in prison meals [34]. The mean all-day purchase-only cost of prison-provided meals and beverages in the GFD was 6.65 ± 0.61 PLN (1.49 ± 0.14 EUR). In Polish supermarkets, this is a purchase price of only 250 g of gluten-free bread or 300 g of gluten-free pasta. Gluten-free (GF) products are more expensive than their standard equivalents [46]. As shown by some data, they may be on average 159% more expensive than regular products in the UK [10] and from 22 to even 334% more expensive in Greece [47]. Probably because of these costs, the menus in all prisons did not include certified GF products; instead, the meals were based on naturally GF products. Both groups of GF products, however, may contain various levels of gluten. Verma et al. [48] showed that its allowable value (20 ppm) was exceeded in 9% of GF products available in stores in Italy.

GFD requires special attention from nutritionists and kitchen staff not only in terms of the nutritional value of the meals served. The difficulties in providing this type of diet in food service establishments are associated with an appropriate supply of GF products, storage of these products, production processes, tools, and processing methods [49]. It has been shown that contamination of kitchen utensils or food-contact surfaces with gluten in school kitchens is promoted by the use of non-protease detergents, lack of rinsing with water immediately before use, storage in open containers, and washing in dishwashers (compared to manual washing) [50]. Therefore, there is a need to investigate GFD served in prisons, with focus on the aspect of proper meal processing in this diet.

Limitations

It should be emphasized that the present results are based solely on analysis of the menus, but they do not include food that prisoners can buy and receive from families. Another limitation in the results is the lack of knowledge of whether all prisoners consume the same portions of meals. This is related to the complicated prison hierarchy and confinement in cells.

5. Conclusions

The results of our research indicate that GFD meals in Polish prisons provide significantly lower amounts of many micronutrients than regular diet meals. This is caused by the exclusion of gluten-containing food from this diet, which is an important source of, e.g., fiber, iron, zinc, and folates. Both analyzed types of diets exhibited excess levels of SFA, sodium, calcium, phosphorus, copper, and vitamins (A, B_6, C, D and folates). The results regarding the supply of nutrients necessitate action from the Central Board of the Prison Service aimed at introduction of external controls and improvement of the quality of meals. There is also a need for a comprehensive discussion on the possibility of supplementation of prisoners, especially with vitamin D. Undoubtedly, the quality of meals is related to the limited financial resources in Polish prisons. This makes it difficult to plan balanced meals by prison nutritionists, especially in the case of GFD meals, which are more expensive.

Author Contributions: Conceptualization, A.K. and P.S.; methodology, A.K., P.S., D.D. and W.G.; software, A.K., P.S. and D.D.; formal analysis, A.K., P.S. and D.D.; data curation, P.S.; writing—original draft preparation, A.K., P.S., D.D. and W.G.; writing—review and editing, A.K. and P.S.; supervision, P.S. and W.G. All authors have read and agreed to the published version of the manuscript.

Funding: This research received no external funding.

Conflicts of Interest: The authors declare no conflict of interest.

References

1. Jasthi, B.; Pettit, J.; Harnack, L. Addition of gluten values to a food and nutrient database. *J. Food Comp. Anal.* **2020**, *85*, 103330. [CrossRef]
2. Henggeler, J.C.; Verissimo, M.; Ramos, F. Non-coeliac gluten sensitivity: A review of the literature. *Trends Food Sci. Technol.* **2017**, *66*, 84–92. [CrossRef]
3. Butterworth, J.; Los, L. Coeliac disease. *Medicine* **2019**, *47*, 314–319. [CrossRef]
4. Ludvigsson, J.F.; Murray, J.A. Epidemiology of celiac disease. *Gastroenterol. Clin. N. Am.* **2019**, *48*, 1–18. [CrossRef]
5. Unalp-Arida, A.; Ruhl, C.E.; Choung, R.S.; Brantner, T.L.; Murray, J.A. Lower prevalence of celiac disease and gluten-related disorders in persons living in southern vs northern latitudes of the United States. *Gastroenterology* **2017**, *152*, 1922–1932. [CrossRef]
6. Australian Institute of Health and Welfare. *The Health of Australia's Prisoners 2018*; Australian Institute of Health and Welfare: Canberra, Australia, 2019. Available online: https://www.aihw.gov.au/getmedia/2e92f007-453d-48a1-9c6b-4c9531cf0371/aihw-phe-246.pdf.aspx?inline=true (accessed on 13 March 2020).
7. Chari, K.A.; Simon, A.E.; DeFrances, C.J.; Maruschak, L. *National Survey of Prison Health Care: Selected Findings*; National Health Statistics Reports; no 96; National Center for Health Statistics: Hyattsville, MD, USA, 2016. Available online: https://www.bjs.gov/content/pub/pdf/nsphcsf.pdf (accessed on 13 March 2020).
8. Central Board of Prison Service in Poland. *Statistical Yearbook for 2019*; Central Board of Prison Service in Poland: Warsaw, Poland, 2020. Available online: https://www.sw.gov.pl/strona/statystyka-roczna (accessed on 3 March 2020). (In Polish)
9. Caio, G.; Volta, U.; Sapone, A.; Leffler, D.A.; De Giorgio, R.; Catassi, C.; Fasano, A. Celiac disease: A comprehensive current review. *BMC Med.* **2019**, *17*, 1–20. [CrossRef] [PubMed]
10. Fry, L.; Madden, A.M.; Fallaize, R. An investigation into the nutritional composition and cost of gluten-free versus regular food products in the UK. *J. Hum. Nutr. Diet.* **2018**, *31*, 108–120. [CrossRef] [PubMed]
11. Martin, J.; Geisel, T.; Maresch, C.; Krieger, K.; Stein, J. Inadequate nutrient intake in patients with celiac disease: Results from a German dietary survey. *Digestion* **2013**, *87*, 240–246. [CrossRef] [PubMed]
12. Shepherd, S.J.; Gibson, P.R. Nutritional inadequacies of the gluten-free diet in both recently diagnosed and long term patients with coeliac disease. *J. Hum. Nutr. Diet.* **2013**, *26*, 349–358. [CrossRef] [PubMed]
13. Hallert, C.; Grant, C.; Grehn, S.; Grännö, C.; Hultén, S.; Midhagen, G.; Ström, M.; Svensson, H.; Valdimarsson, T. Evidence of poor vitamin status in coeliac patients on a gluten-free diet for 10 years. *Aliment. Pharmacol. Ther.* **2002**, *16*, 1333–1339. [CrossRef]

14. Skodje, G.I.; Minelle, I.H.; Rolfsen, K.L.; Iacovou, M.; Lundin, K.E.A.; Veierød, M.B.; Henriksen, C. Dietary and symptom assessment in adults with self-reported non-coeliac gluten sensitivity. *Clin. Nutr. ESPEN* **2019**, *31*, 88–94. [CrossRef] [PubMed]
15. Salazar Quero, J.C.; Espín Jaime, B.; Rodríguez Martínez, A.; Argüelles Martín, F.; García Jiménez, R.; Rubio Murillo, M.; Pizarro Martín, A. Nutritional assessment of gluten-free diet. Is gluten-free diet deficient in some nutrient? *An. Pediatr. Engl. Ed.* **2015**, *83*, 33–39. [CrossRef] [PubMed]
16. Wild, D.; Robins, G.G.; Burley, V.J.; Howdle, P.D. Evidence of high sugar intake, and low fibre and mineral intake, in the gluten-free diet. *Aliment. Pharmacol. Ther.* **2010**, *32*, 573–581. [CrossRef]
17. Gobbetti, M.; Pontonio, E.; Filannino, P.; Rizzello, C.G.; De Angelis, M.; Di Cagno, R. How to improve the gluten-free diet: The state of the art from a food science perspective. *Food Res. Int.* **2018**, *110*, 22–32. [CrossRef] [PubMed]
18. Rozporządzenie Ministra Sprawiedliwości z dn. 19 Lutego 2016 r. w Sprawie Wyżywienia Osadzonych w Zakładach Karnych i Aresztach Śledczych [Regulation of the Minister of Justice of 19 February 2016 on Nutrition of Polish Prisoners]. Available online: http://isap.sejm.gov.pl/isap.nsf/download.xsp/WDU20160000302/O/D20160302.pdf (accessed on 25 March 2020). (In Polish)
19. Ustawa z Dnia 6 Czerwca 1997 r.—Kodeks Karny Wykonawczy [Act of 6 June 1997—Executive Penal Code]. Dz. U. 1997 Nr 90 Poz. 557. Available online: http://isap.sejm.gov.pl/isap.nsf/DocDetails.xsp?id=WDU19970900557 (accessed on 25 March 2020). (In Polish)
20. Kunachowicz, H.; Przygoda, B.; Nadolna, I.; Iwanow, K. *Tabele Składu i Wartości Odżywczych Żywności [Tables of Composition and Nutritional Value of Food Products]*; PZWL: Warsaw, Poland, 2017. (In Polish)
21. FoodData Central. Available online: https://fdc.nal.usda.gov/fdc-app.html#/ (accessed on 25 March 2020).
22. Jarosz, M. *Human Nutrition Recommendation for Polish Population*; Food and Nutrition Institute: Warsaw, Poland, 2017. (In Polish)
23. Soto, L.G.; Martín-Masot, R.; Nestares, T.; Maldonado, J. Analysis of the gluten-free menus served in school canteens: Are they balanced? *Nutr. Hosp.* **2019**, *36*, 912–918. (In Spanish) [CrossRef]
24. Laskowski, W.; Górska-Warsewicz, H.; Rejman, K.; Czeczotko, M.; Zwolińska, J. How important are cereals and cereal products in the average polish diet? *Nutrients* **2019**, *11*, 679. [CrossRef]
25. Jaworska, A. Aktywność fizyczna w zakładach karnych a podstawowe wymiary osobowości mężczyzn odbywających karę pozbawienia wolności [Physical activity in prisons and the basic dimensions of personality of men serving prison sentences]. *Pol. J. Soc. Rehabil.* **2015**, *9*, 137–157. (In Polish)
26. Kosendiak, A.; Trzeciak, D. Motywy i czynniki warunkujące poziom aktywności fizycznej aresztowanych oraz skazanych w warunkach izolacji [Motives and factors conditioning the level of physical activity arrested and convicted people in isolation conditions]. *Roz. Nauk. AWF Wroc.* **2019**, *64*, 70–80. (In Polish)
27. Dall'Asta, C.; Scarlato, A.P.; Galaverna, G.; Brighenti, F.; Pellegrini, N. Dietary exposure to fumonisins and evaluation of nutrient intake in a group of adult celiac patients on a gluten-free diet. *Mol. Nutr. Food Res.* **2012**, *56*, 632–640. [CrossRef]
28. Miranda, J.; Lasa, A.; Bustamante, M.A.; Churruca, I.; Simon, E. Nutritional differences between a gluten-free diet and a diet containing equivalent products with gluten. *Plant Foods Hum. Nutr.* **2014**, *69*, 182–187. [CrossRef]
29. Thompson, T.; Dennis, M.; Higgins, L.A.; Lee, A.R.; Sharrett, K. Gluten-free diet survey: Are Americans with coeliac disease consuming recommended amounts of fibre, iron, calcium and grain foods? *J. Hum. Nutr. Diet.* **2005**, *18*, 163–169. [CrossRef] [PubMed]
30. Roy, P.; Orikasa, T.; Okadome, H.; Nakamura, N.; Shiina, T. Processing conditions, rice properties, health and environment. *Int. J. Environ. Res. Public Health* **2011**, *8*, 1957–1976. [CrossRef]
31. Aaltonen, K.; Laurikka, P.; Huhtala, H.; Mäki, M.; Kaukinen, K.; Kurppa, K. The long-term consumption of oats in celiac disease patients is safe: A large cross-sectional study. *Nutrients* **2017**, *9*, 611. [CrossRef]
32. Polish Association of People with Celiac Disease and the Gluten-Free Diet. Available online: https://celiakia.pl/produkty-dozwolone/ (accessed on 8 September 2020). (In Polish).

33. Rozporządzenie Ministra Sprawiedliwości z dnia 2 Września 2003 roku w Sprawie Określenia Wartości Dziennej Normy Wyżywienia oraz Rodzaju diet Wydawanych Osobom Osadzonym w Zakładach Karnych i Aresztach Śledczych. [Regulation of the Minister of Justice of 2 September 2003 on Nutritional Value of Daily Food Rations and Type of Diets Served in Prisons and Detention Centers]. Available online: http://isap.sejm.gov.pl/isap.nsf/download.xsp/WDU20031671633/O/D20031633.pdf (accessed on 21 July 2020). (In Polish)
34. Stanikowski, P.; Michalak-Majewska, M.; Domagała, D.; Jabłońska-Ryś, E.; Sławińska, A. Implementation of dietary reference intake standards in prison menus in Poland. *Nutrients* **2020**, *12*, 728. [CrossRef] [PubMed]
35. Łazarczyk, M.; Grabańska-Martyńska, K.; Cymerys, M. Analiza spożycia soli kuchennej u pacjentów z nadciśnieniem tętniczym [The analysis of salt consumption in patients with hypertension]. *Forum Zab. Metabol.* **2016**, *7*, 84–92. (In Polish)
36. Micic, D.; Rao, V.L.; Semrad, C.E. Celiac disease and its role in the development of metabolic bone disease. *J. Clin. Densitom.* **2020**, *23*, 190–199. [CrossRef]
37. Sattgast, L.H.; Gallo, S.; Frankenfeld, C.L.; Moshfegh, A.J.; Slavin, M. Nutritional intake and bone health among adults with probable undiagnosed, untreated celiac disease: What we eat in America and NHANES 2009–2014. *J. Am. Coll. Nutr.* **2020**, *39*, 112–121. [CrossRef]
38. Kinsey, L.; Burden, S.T.; Bannerman, E. A dietary survey to determine if patients with coeliac disease are meeting current healthy heating guidelines and how their diet compares to that of the British general population. *Eur. J. Clin. Nutr.* **2008**, *62*, 1333–1342. [CrossRef]
39. Calvo, M.S.; Tucker, K.L. Is phosphorus intake that exceeds dietary requirements a risk factor in bone health? *Ann. N. Y. Acad. Sci.* **2013**, *1301*, 29–35. [CrossRef]
40. Kucharska, E.; Seidler, T.; Balejko, E.; Bogacka, A.; Gryza, M.; Szczuko, M. Porównanie całodziennych jadłospisów osadzonych w niektórych aresztach śledczych i zakładach karnych [Comparison of daily dietary rations in some court detention houses and prisons]. *Bromatol. Chem. Toksykol.* **2009**, *42*, 36–44. (In Polish)
41. Kucharska, A.; Gronau, M.; Sińska, B.; Michota-Katulska, E.; Zegan, M. Ocena realizacji zaleceń żywieniowych dla osób osadzonych na przykładzie wybranego aresztu śledczego [Assessment of the implementation of dietary guidelines for inmates in a selected detention center]. *Probl. Hig. Epidemiol.* **2013**, *94*, 807–810. (In Polish)
42. Waśkiewicz, A.; Sygnowska, E.; Broda, G. Dietary intake of vitamins B_6, B_{12} and folate in relation to homocysteine serum concentration in the adult Polish population—WOBASZ Project. *Kardiol. Pol.* **2010**, *68*, 275–282.
43. Vici, G.; Camilletti, D.; Polzonetti, V. Possible role of vitamin D in celiac disease onset. *Nutrients* **2020**, *12*, 1051. [CrossRef]
44. Nwosu, B.U.; Maranda, L.; Berry, R.; Colocino, B.; Flores, C.D., Sr.; Folkman, K.; Groblewski, T.; Ruze, P. The vitamin D status of prison inmates. *PLoS ONE* **2014**, *9*, e90623. [CrossRef]
45. Jacobs, E.T.; Mullany, C.J. Vitamin D deficiency and inadequacy in a correctional population. *Nutrition* **2015**, *31*, 659–663. [CrossRef]
46. Singh, J.; Whelan, K. Limited availability and higher cost of gluten-free foods. *J. Hum. Nutr. Diet.* **2011**, *24*, 479–486. [CrossRef]
47. Panagiotou, S.; Kontogianni, M.D. The economic burden of gluten-free products and gluten-free diet: A cost estimation analysis in Greece. *J. Hum. Nutr. Diet.* **2017**, *30*, 746–752. [CrossRef]
48. Verma, A.K.; Gatti, S.; Galeazzi, T.; Monachesi, C.; Padella, L.; Del Baldo, G.; Annibali, R.; Lionetti, E.; Catassi, C. Gluten contamination in naturally or labeled gluten-free products marketed in Italy. *Nutrients* **2017**, *9*, 115. [CrossRef]
49. Bioletti, L.; Capuano, M.T.; Vietti, F.; Cesari, L.; Emma, L.; Leggio, K.; Fransos, L.; Marzullo, A.; Ropolo, S.; Strumia, C. Celiac disease and school food service in Piedmont Region: Evaluation of gluten-free meal. *Ann. Ig.* **2016**, *28*, 145–157. [CrossRef]
50. Galan-Malo, P.; Oritz, J.-C.; Carrascon, V.; Razquin, P.; Mata, L. A study to reduce the allergen contamination in food-contact surfaces at canteen kitchens. *Int. J. Gastron. Food Sci.* **2019**, *17*, 100165. [CrossRef]

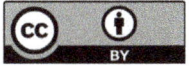

© 2020 by the authors. Licensee MDPI, Basel, Switzerland. This article is an open access article distributed under the terms and conditions of the Creative Commons Attribution (CC BY) license (http://creativecommons.org/licenses/by/4.0/).

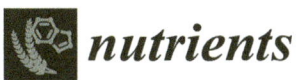

Article

Updated Food Composition Database for Cereal-Based Gluten Free Products in Spain: Is Reformulation Moving on?

Violeta Fajardo, María Purificación González *, María Martínez,
María de Lourdes Samaniego-Vaesken, María Achón, Natalia Úbeda [†] and Elena Alonso-Aperte [†]

Departamento de Ciencias Farmacéuticas y de la Salud, Facultad de Farmacia, Universidad San Pablo-CEU, CEU Universities, Urbanización Montepríncipe, Alcorcón, 28925 Madrid, Spain;
violeta.fajardomartin@ceu.es (V.F.); mar.martinez1.ce@ceindo.ceu.es (M.M.); l.samaniego@ceu.es (M.d.L.S.-V.); achontu@ceu.es (M.A.); nubeda@ceu.es (N.Ú.); eaperte@ceu.es (E.A.-A.)
* Correspondence: mpgonzal@ceu.es; Tel.: +34-913-724-719
[†] Natalia Úbeda and Elena Alonso-Aperte share senior authorship.

Received: 21 July 2020; Accepted: 5 August 2020; Published: 7 August 2020

Abstract: We developed a comprehensive composition database of 629 cereal-based gluten free (GF) products available in Spain. Information on ingredients and nutritional composition was retrieved from food package labels. GF products were primarily composed of rice and/or corn flour, and 90% of them included added rice starch. The most common added fat was sunflower oil (present in one third of the products), followed by palm fat, olive oil, and cocoa. Only 24.5% of the products had the nutrition claim "no added sugar". Fifty-six percent of the GF products had sucrose in their formulation. Xanthan gum was the most frequently employed fiber, appearing in 34.2% of the GF products, followed by other commonly used such as hydroxypropyl methylcellulose (23.1%), guar gum (19.7%), and vegetable gums (19.6%). Macronutrient analysis revealed that 25.4% of the products could be labeled as a source of fiber. Many of the considered GF food products showed very high contents of energy (33.5%), fats (28.5%), saturated fatty acids (30.0%), sugars (21.6%), and salt (28.3%). There is a timid reformulation in fat composition and salt reduction, but a lesser usage of alternative flours and pseudocereals.

Keywords: gluten-free products; celiac disease; gluten-free diet; gluten containing products; food composition database

---

1. Introduction

One percent of the general population in the Western world is affected by celiac disease (CD), one of the most common food intolerances in Europe [1]. CD is an autoimmune disorder with an aberrant response to gluten proteins with subsequent atrophy of intestinal villi, impaired intestinal absorption, and malnutrition. Extra-intestinal symptoms such as fatigue, iron deficiency, and neurological/psychological disorders (e.g., depression) may also be present. Long-term risks associated with CD, such as lymphoma, osteoporosis, and anemia, have also been reported [2].

A strict and lifelong adherence to a gluten free diet (GFD) is the first-line treatment and, currently, the only effective therapy for celiac patients and all other gluten related disorders, such as non-celiac gluten sensitivity or wheat allergy [3]. Gluten originates from a family of proteins found in wheat (gliadins and glutenins), rye (secalins), barley (hordeins), and oats (avenins), or in their hybridized strains (e.g., spelt or kamut) [4]. A GFD comprises only naturally gluten free (GF) food products (e.g., legumes, fruit and vegetables, unprocessed meat, fish, eggs, dairy products, and GF cereals, such as rice or corn) and/or substitutes of wheat-based foods, specially manufactured without gluten or having a gluten content lower than 20 ppm, as per European legislation [5]. For the traditional gluten-containing foods, such as bakery products, there is currently a wide variety of GF options available that use GF cereals (rice, corn, millet, and sorghum) and pseudocereals (quinoa, buckwheat, amaranth, and teff) as their base ingredients [6]. However, a GFD is difficult to follow because gluten is an ingredient widely used in the food industry, appearing in products that originally do not contain gluten such as meat, fish, and many other foodstuffs [7]. Hence, product labels and ingredient lists need to be carefully reviewed.

Consumer's interest and demand has led to a significant increase in the production and sales of GF products. Global market data indicate that GF product sales are forecasted to increase by a compound annual growth rate of 7.6% between 2020 and 2027 [8]. In the last decade, Spain has been the leader country increasing its production of GF goods (18.8%), compared to Western Europe and the rest of the world (13.6% and 15.4%, respectively), and has become the third world producer of this type of products, after U.S.A. and Brazil. In 2019, the European region held the maximum market share in the GF products market [7]. Reasons for this growth are not only due to purchases by those with CD or those with a gluten sensitivity but are also propelled by changes in consumer attitudes towards health. Mainstream consumers are experimenting with their diets for health-related reasons, and "free-from" foods (such as GF foods) are part of that trend [9].

However, comprehensive nutritional composition data of GF products, mainly vitamin and mineral content, are still scarce or limited [10,11]. More importantly, access to such data is even more restricted, since there is a broad lack of micronutrient data in food composition tables, databases, and food labels. This statement warrants the need of providing new data on mineral and vitamins in GF food products, to complete food composition tables or databases, to cover regulatory purposes, and/or to assess population dietary intakes [12]. Composition data are useful to evaluate the adequacy of nutrient intake of celiac patients, on which the debate is still open, and are, therefore, strongly needed [13].

The GFD has demonstrated benefits in managing some gluten-related disorders, although nutritional imbalances have been reported. Although a GFD is associated with being healthier by some authors [9,14], epidemiological studies indicate nutritional imbalances in different celiac populations following a GFD, both in children [13,15] and in adults [16,17]. They refer to both macronutrients and micronutrients, including minerals. Overall, nutritional imbalances include high lipid, high protein, and low fiber intakes, and lack of adequacy to reference intakes of vitamin D, calcium, and magnesium [13,15]. Celiac patients may also be at risk of iron and folate deficiencies [17]. Some authors state that nutritional deficiencies in CD patients may be due to GF products, which are made with highly refined flours and high amounts of fat and sugar to achieve a texture resembling the typical and unique viscoelastic properties of wheat [18,19].

To provide better consumer information, the objective of this paper is to develop a nutritional food composition database including cereal-based GF products available in Spain. For this purpose, we estimated the nutritional composition of the products considering both the nutritional information and the ingredients reported on the product label, focusing on the critical components that define the nutritional quality of a GFD (added flours, starches, fats, sugars, and fiber).

2. Materials and Methods

2.1. Design and Data Collection

The present study involved the compilation of cereal-based gluten-free (GF) products available in the Spanish market. Products and brands were gathered systematically from manufacturer websites and/or specialized retail stores and supermarkets with the highest market shares in Spain between September 2016 and March 2019. Retailers such as Carrefour, Hipercor, Mercadona, Alcampo, and Lidl, as well as smaller specialized stores, were visited. Information on ingredients and nutritional composition was retrieved from the food package labels. Major commercial and distribution brands were selected. All products included in the study showed one of the following claims on the package: the European Crossed Grain Trademark, the Spanish Federation of Coeliac Associations (FACE) crossed grain symbol, or the "gluten free" claim.

2.2. Food Database Development

The cereal-based GF food database was developed according to LanguaL™ Thesaurus EuroFIR [20]. In total, 629 cereal-based GF food items were categorized into four groups, nine subgroups, and thirteen subgroup categories in the developed database, in consonance with the LanguaL™ classification. The four groups were beverages, milk, milk product, or milk substitutes, grain or grain products, and miscellaneous food products.

The grain or grain products group comprised six subgroups: bread and similar, breakfast cereals, cereal or cereal-like milling products and derivatives, fine bakery ware, pasta and similar products, and savory cereal dishes. Beverages (non-milk) included alcoholic beverages. The milk, milk product, or milk substitutes group included data from frozen dairy desserts. Finally, miscellaneous food products involved prepared food products.

Each cereal-based GF food item was assigned to one of the following subgroups and categories: beer or beer-like beverages, frozen dairy desserts, bread products, leavened breads, unleavened breads, crisp breads, and rusks, breakfast cereals and cereal bars, cereal or cereal-like milling products and derivatives, biscuits, sweets, and semi-sweets, pancakes or waffles, pastries and cakes, pasta and similar products, pasta dishes, pies, unsweetened, or pizzas, savory cereal dishes, and savory snacks (see Table 1). Bread products included breadcrumbs. Leavened breads included rolls, buns, breads baked in pans and French type. Cereal or cereal-like milling products and derivatives included flour and flour preparations for baking products.

2.3. Food Composition in Terms of Ingredients

The ingredient list used in the formulation of the GF products was analyzed. Four groups of critical ingredients were considered: starchy ingredients (i.e., flour or starch), fats (oils and fats), sugars (i.e., dextrose), and added fibers (i.e., xanthan gum). Ingredients were chosen according to their impact on the nutritional profile of GF products. In each case, the top ten most frequently used ingredients were considered.

2.4. Nutritional Information Study

The nutritional composition of each product item included in the database is given in terms of quantity of energy and nutrients per 100 g of product as sold. Energy expressed in kcal, macronutrients (fats (g), saturated fatty acids (g), carbohydrates (g), sugars (g), protein (g)), fiber (g), and salt (g) were the data on nutrient composition reported on the label of each product. Micronutrients, vitamin, and mineral contents were not declared on the label in hardly any GF products.

2.5. Statistical Analysis

Descriptive data on ingredients are expressed as frequency (number of products including a specific ingredient and percentage based on the total products within the category or the subgroup). Data on nutrient composition are expressed as average and standard deviation.

3. Results

GF products available in Spanish markets were systematically compiled between September 2016 and March 2019. In total, 629 cereal-based GF products were studied, and each food item was assigned to one of nine subgroups, based on LanguaL™ Thesaurus 2017 (Figure 1).

The main group was fine bakery ware ($n = 229$; 36.4%), followed by bread and similar products ($n = 152$; 24.2%) and pasta and similar products ($n = 88$; 13.9%). Minor categories were alcoholic beverages (*n* = 14; 2.2%) and frozen dairy desserts (*n* = 6; 0.9%). The targeted GF products belonged to more than 70 different commercial brands. Among the top five manufacturers of GF products (Schär, Santiveri, Airos, Adpan, and Proceli), four of them are Spanish companies. However, it should be noted that the leading producers were mostly different across different GF product categories. We developed an initial GF product database in 2016, including 271 cereal-based GF food products. Up to 10% of the foodstuffs found in the present update are no longer available, and 24.5% have been reformulated.

The database is available for research purposes on demand.

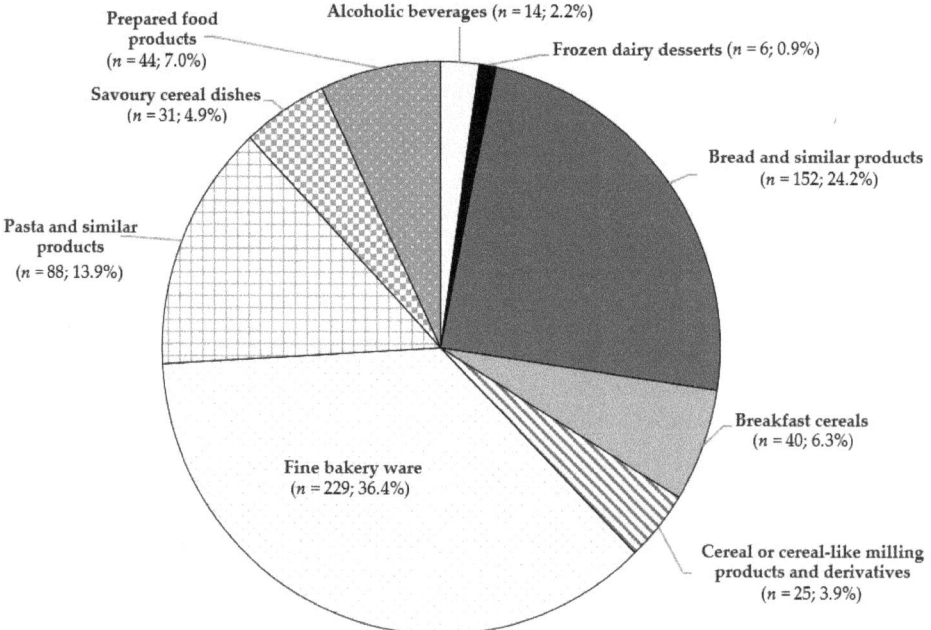

Figure 1. Cereal-based gluten free (GF) products included in the database (*n* = 629).

3.1. Food Composition in Terms of Ingredients

Cereal-based GF products were primarily composed of rice and/or corn flour, and almost 90% of them included added rice starch (Tables 1 and 2). Less than 10% of the GF products were formulated with other kinds of flours, such as buckwheat, soy and other legumes, brown rice, millet, or quinoa. Oatmeal, sorghum, amaranth, teff, guar, chia, chestnut, flax, or potato flours were very rarely present in the ingredient list. Corn starch was present in the formulation of 60% of the products, and other commonly added were rice and potato starches. Tapioca starch, modified starch, and potato maltodextrin were also found in some products. Barley malt was the main cereal used for beer-like beverages.

Considering bread products, wheat is the main flour used in Spain, but it must be substituted by rice flour, followed by corn flour, and frequently added with rice or corn starches when baking GF breads. Corn flour is more frequently used than rice flour when preparing GF breakfast cereals, pasta, and savory snacks. Soya flour was most frequently used in fine bakery ware, with 26% of biscuits, sweets, and semi-sweets containing this type of flour. Added starches were found in all products except for breakfast cereals and beer-like beverages.

Table 1. Types of flour used in the formulation of gluten free (GF) products.

Food Groups	Food Subgroups (n)	Rice n (%)	Corn * n (%)	Brown Rice n (%)	Millet n (%)	Buckwheat n (%)	Soy n (%)	Other Legumes ** n (%)	Quinoa n (%)	Barley Malt n (%)	Other Flours *** n (%)
Beverages (non-milk)	Alcoholic beverages (14)	2 (14.3)	5 (35.7)	0	1 (7.1)	0	0	0	0	10 (71.4)	0
	Beer or beer-like beverages (14)	2 (14.3)	5 (35.7)	0	1 (7.1)	0	0	0	0	10 (71.4)	0
Milk, milk product, or milk substitutes	Frozen dairy desserts (6)	4 (66.6)	2 (33.3)	0	0	0	1 (16.7)	4 (66.7)	0	0	0
	Bread and similar (152)	88 (57.9)	36 (23.7)	13 (8.6)	22 (14.5)	22 (14.5)	3 (2.0)	15 (9.9)	10 (6.6)	0	18 (11.8)
	Bread products (11)	4 (36.4)	5 (45.5)	0	1 (9.1)	1 (9.1)	1 (9.1)	0	0	0	0
	Leavened breads (89)	50 (56.2)	12 (13.5)	7 (7.9)	19 (2.1)	11 (12.4)	2 (2.2)	7 (7.9)	8 (9.0)	0	10 (11.2)
	Unleavened breads, crisp breads, and rusks (52)	34 (65.4)	19 (36.5)	6 (11.5)	2 (3.8)	10 (19.2)	0	8 (15.4)	2 (3.8)	0	8 (15.4)
	Breakfast cereals (40)	18 (45.0)	29 (72.5)	1 (15.5)	2 (5.0)	4 (10.0)	1	0	4 (10.0)	0	10 (25.0)
	Breakfast cereals (35)	15 (42.9)	26 (74.3)	1 (2.9)	0	3 (8.6)	1 (2.9)	0	4 (11.4)	0	8 (22.9)
	Cereal bars (5)	3 (60.0)	3 (60.0)	0	2 (40.0)	1 (20.0)	0	0	0	0	2 (40.0)
Grain or grain products	Cereal or cereal-like milling products and derivatives (25)	11 (44.0)	11 (44.0)	1 (4.0)	0	2 (8.0)	0	3 (12.0)	0	0	2 (8.0)
	Fine bakery ware (229)	99 (43.2)	80 (34.9)	7 (3.1)	5 (2.2)	7 (3.1)	42 (18.3)	20 (8.7)	0	0	9 3.9)
	Biscuits, sweets, and semi-sweets (96)	57 (59.4)	64 (66.7)	1 (1.0)	5 (5.2)	3 (3.1)	25 (26.0)	8 (8.3)	0	0	10 (10.4)
	Pancakes or waffles (6)	0	0	0	0	1 (16.7)	0	1 (16.7)	0	0	0
	Pastries and cakes (127)	42 (33.1)	16 (94.1)	6 (4.7)	0	3 (2.4)	17 (13.4)	11 (8.7)	7 (8.0)	0	2 (2.3)
	Pasta and similar products (88)	54 (61.4)	81 (92.0)	9 (10.2)	7 (7.9)	4 (4.5)	0	1 (1.1)	0	0	0
	Savory cereal dishes (31)	19 (61.3)	19 (61.3)	1 (3.2)	2 (6.5)	8 (25.8)	2 (6.5)	2 (6.5)	0	0	1 (3.2)
	Pasta dishes (13)	8 (61.5)	8 (61.5)	0	1 (7.7)	0	2 (15.4)	2 (15.4)	0	0	0
	Pies, unsweetened, or pizzas (18)	11 (61.1)	11 (61.1)	1 (5.6)	1 (5.6)	8 (44.4)	0	0	0	0	1 (5.6)
	Prepared food products (44)	10 (22.7)	20 (45.5)	9 (20.5)	0	0	4 (9.1)	1 (2.3)	5 (11.4)	0	0
Miscellaneous food products	Savory cereal dishes (16)	6 (37.5)	4 (25.0)	0	0	0	0	0	0	0	0
	Savory snacks (28)	4 (14.3)	16 (57.1)	9 (32.1)	0	0	4 (14.3)	1 (3.6)	5 (17.9)	0	0
	Total (629)	305 (48.5)	283 (45.0)	41 (6.5)	39 (6.2)	47 (7.5)	53 (8.4)	46 (7.3)	26 (4.1)	10 (1.6)	43 (6.8)

Results are expressed as frequency (n, number of products including a specific ingredient) and (percentage based on the total products within the category or the subgroup). * Includes corn flour, corn grits, or corn. ** Other legumes include chickpea, pea, carob, lentil, lupine, or fava bean. *** Other flours include oatmeal, sorghum, amaranth, teff, guar, chia, chestnut, flax, or potato.

Table 2. Types of starch used in the formulation of gluten free (GF) products.

Food Groups	Food Subgroups (n)	Corn n (%)	Rice n (%)	Potato n (%)	Tapioca n (%)	Modified n (%)	Modified Corn n (%)	Modified Tapioca n (%)	Modified Potato n (%)	Potato Maltodextrin n (%)	Wheat Starch without Gluten n (%)
Beverages (non-milk)	Alcoholic beverages (14)	0	0	0	0	0	0	0	0	0	0
	Beer or beer-like beverages (14)	0	0	0	0	0	0	0	0	0	0
Milk, milk product, or milk substitutes	Frozen dairy desserts (6)	3 (50.0)	1 (16.7)	1 (16.7)	0	0	0	0	0	0	0
	Bread and similar (152)	134 (88.2)	33 (21.7)	17 (11.2)	18 (11.8)	1 (0.7)	2 (1.3)	0	0	0	1 (0.7)
	Bread products (11)	10 (90.9)	0	0	1 (9.1)	0	0	0	0	0	0
	Leavened breads (89)	85 (95.5)	28 (31.5)	4 (4.5)	15 (16.9)	1 (1.1)	0	0	0	0	0
	Unleavened breads, crisp breads, and rusks (52)	39 (75.0)	5 (9.6)	13 (25.0)	2 (3.8)	0	2 (3.8)	0	0	0	1 (1.9)
	Breakfast cereals (40)	0	0	0	0	0	0	0	0	0	0
	Breakfast cereals (35)	0	0	0	0	0	0	0	0	0	0
	Cereal bars (5)	0	0	0	0	0	0	0	0	0	0
Grain or grain products	Cereal or cereal-like milling products and derivatives (25)	17 (68.0)	1 (4.0)	4 (16.0)	3 (12.0)	1 (4.0)	0	0	0	0	0
	Fine bakery ware (229)	182 (79.5)	58 (25.3)	74 (32.3)	14 (6.1)	5 (2.2)	16 (7.0)	11 (4.8)	1 (0.4)	6 (2.6)	4 (1.7)
	Biscuits, sweets, and semi-sweets (96)	64 (66.7)	26 (27.1)	46 (47.9)	2 (2.1)	0	12 (12.5)	11 (11.5)	1 (1.0)	6 (6.3)	0
	Pancakes or waffles (6)	6 (100)	0	0	0	0	0	0	0	0	1 (16.7)
	Pastries and cakes (127)	112 (88.2)	32 (25.2)	28 (22.0)	12 (9.4)	5 (3.9)	4 (3.1)	0	0	0	3 (2.4)
	Pasta and similar products (88)	2 (2.3)	0	4 (4.5)	0	0	0	0	0	0	0
	Savory cereal dishes (31)	19 (61.3)	10 (32.3)	7 (22.6)	0	6 (19.4)	2 (6.5)	0	0	0	7 (22.6)
	Pasta dishes (13)	12 (92.3)	3 (23.1)	4 (30.8)	0	3 (23.1)	1 (7.7)	0	0	0	0
	Pies, unsweetened, or pizzas (18)	7 (38.9)	7 (38.9)	3 (16.7)	0	3 (16.7)	1 (5.6)	0	0	0	7 (38.9)
	Prepared food products (44)	20 (45.5)	2 (4.5)	11 (2.3)	2 (4.5)	2 (4.5)	4 (9.1)	4 (9.1)	0	0	0
Miscellaneous food products	Savory cereal dishes (16)	12 (75.0)	1 (6.3)	9 (56.3)	2 (12.5)	2 (33.3)	2 (12.5)	0	0	0	0
	Savory snacks (28)	8 (28.6)	1 (3.6)	2 (7.1)	0	0	2 (7.1)	4 (14.3)	0	0	0
Total (629)		377 (59.9)	105 (16.7)	118 (18.7)	37 (5.9)	15 (2.4)	24 (3.8)	15 (2.4)	1 (0.2)	6 (1.0)	12 (1.9)

Results are expressed as frequency (n, number of products including a specific ingredient) and (percentage based on the total products within the category or the subgroup).

One hundred thirty different combinations of added fats were found in the recorded GF food products. The most added fat was sunflower oil, which was present in almost one third of the products, followed by palm fat, olive oil, and cocoa, all used similarly in around 13% of the products. Other animal fats (butter, cream, or lard), margarines, rapeseed oil, and coconut oil were more seldom used (Table 3). Therefore, unsaturated fats were predominant in most of the GF foodstuffs considered in the database. However, palm fat was the main fat added to biscuits, sweets, and semi-sweets, classified in the fine bakery ware subgroup, in addition to other saturated fats such as cocoa and animal fats. When focusing on frozen dairy desserts, it was observed that only saturated fats were present (animal fats, coconut oil, palm oil, and cocoa). Both results are in accordance with the high amounts of fat and saturated fats found, respectively, in the subgroups in the macronutrient analysis (see Section 3.2). The three most used margarines were made by: palm, coconut, and sunflower; palm, coconut, and rapeseed; and coconut with sunflower. Bread and similar products and fine bakery ware were the subgroups in which margarines were more frequently used. Taken together, palm fat and margarines made up with palm oil were present in 22.8% of the GF products. Finally, no added fats or oils were used as ingredients in pasta and similar products, according to the labeling.

Only 154 GF foodstuffs (24.5%) had the nutrition claim "no added sugar" on the label [21], being pasta and similar products the most representative subgroup of this fact (Table 4). Among the added sugars, we found that 55.8 % of the GF products had sucrose in their formulation. Other sugars and sweeteners less employed were, in order of frequency, glucose, fructose, dextrose, and lactose. Other rich sugar ingredients such us non-refined or cane sugar, rice syrup, beetroot sugar syrup, and honey were also present in the GF products. Leavened breads, biscuits, sweets, semi-sweets, pastries, and cakes were the subgroups were GF products more frequently contained added sugars, with almost 100% of the products containing sucrose, dextrose or glucose, and fructose. Very few breakfast cereals and fine bakery ware (<3%) included no calorie sweeteners.

Table 5 shows the type of fibers used in the formulation of GF products. Xanthan gum was the most frequently employed fiber, appearing in 34.2% of the GF products, followed by other commonly used such as hydroxypropyl methyl cellulose (23.1%), guar gum (19.7%), vegetable gums (psyllium, bamboo, chicory, potato, rice, pea, corn, etc.) (19.6%), and sodium carboxymethyl cellulose (6.4%). Fibers less frequently found in GF products were citrus fiber, carrageenan, pectin, cellulose, locust bean gum, and apple fiber (appearing in 1.6 to 2.7% of the products). The least fiber enriched products were breakfast cereals and pasta and similar products, whereas the most frequently supplemented were bread and similar products, fine bakery ware, and savory cereal dishes. Macronutrient analysis (Table 6) revealed that 25.4% of the products could be labeled as a source of fiber (>3 g/100 g), mostly breads, breakfast cereals, milling products, and fine bakery ware.

3.2. Nutritional Information

The highest amount of energy, total fats and sugars was found in the fine bakery ware subgroup (426.1 ± 77.7 kcal/100 g, 20.5 ± 6.8 g/100 g and 22.2 ± 9.2 g/100 g, respectively). The highest content of saturated fats was found in frozen dairy desserts (8.8 ± 4.2 g/100 g); proteins in savory cereal dishes (7.7 ± 2.0 g/100 g); carbohydrates in pasta and similar products (76.5 ± 5.9 g/100 g); and fiber and salt in bread and similar products (5.2 ± 2.2 g/100 g, 1.5 ± 0.5 g/100 g, respectively). Average salt content in all products was 0.6 ± 0.4 g/100 g. Highest contents were found in bread and similar products, savory cereal dishes, and prepared food products (Table 6).

Table 3. Fat ingredients used in the formulation of gluten free (GF) products.

Food Groups	Food Subgroups (n)	Sunflower Oil n (%)	Palm Fat * n (%)	Olive Oil n (%)	Cocoa n (%)	Animal Fats (Butter, Cream or Lard) n (%)	Margarine 1 (Palm, Coconut and Sunflower) n (%)	Rapeseed Oil n (%)	Coconut Oil n (%)	Margarine 2 (Palm, Coconut and Rapeseed) n (%)	Margarine 3 (Coconut and Sunflower) n (%)
Beverages (non-milk)	Alcoholic beverages (14)	0	0	0	0	0	0	0	0	0	0
	Beer or beer-like beverages (14)	0	0	0	0	0	0	0	0	0	0
Milk, milk product, or milk substitutes	Frozen dairy desserts (6)	0	2 (33.3)	0	2 (33.3)	4 (66.7)	0	0	3 (50)	0	0
	Bread and similar (152)	57 (37.5)	7 (4.6)	23 (15.1)	1 (0.7)	0	18 (11.8)	9 (5.9)	1 (0.7)	0	12 (7.9)
	Bread products (11)	0	1 (9.1)	2 (18.2)	0	0	0	0	0	0	0
	Leavened breads (89)	45 (50.6)	1 (1.1)	12 (13.5)	1 (1.1)	0	14 (15.7)	3 (3.4)	0	0	10 (11.2)
	Unleavened breads, crisp breads, and rusks (52)	12 (23.1)	5 (9.6)	9 (17.3)	0	0	4 (7.7)	6 (11.5)	1 (1.9)	0	2 (3.8)
	Breakfast cereals (40)	9 (22.5)	6 (15.0)	0	5 (12.5)	1 (2.5)	0	1 (2.5)	1 (2.5)	0	0
	Breakfast cereals (35)	6 (17.1)	4 (11.4)	0	3 (8.6)	0	0	1 (2.9)	1 (2.9)	0	0
	Cereal bars (5)	3 (60.0)	2 (40.0)	0	2 (40.0)	1 (20.0)	0	0	0	0	0
Grain or grain products	Cereal or cereal-like milling products and derivatives (25)	0	0	0	0	0	0	0	0	0	0
	Fine bakery ware (229)	98 (42.8)	61 (26.6)	35 (15.3)	68 (29.7)	41 (17.9)	11 (4.8)	8 (3.5)	16 (7.0)	18 (7.9)	8 (3.5)
	Biscuits, sweets, and semi-sweets (96)	22 (22.9)	38 (39.6)	21 (21.9)	24 (25.0)	10 (10.4)	3 (3.1)	4 (4.2)	11 (11.4)	14 (14.6)	0
	Pancakes or waffles (6)	1 (16.7)	0	0	0	4 (66.7)	0	0	0	0	0
	Pastries and cakes (127)	75 (59.1)	23 (18.1)	14 (11.0)	44 (34.6)	27 (21.2)	8 (6.3)	4 (3.1)	5 (3.9)	4 (3.1)	8 (6.3)
	Pasta and similar products (88)	0	0	0	0	0	0	0	0	0	0
	Savory cereal dishes (31)	19 (61.3)	4 (12.9)	13 (41.9)	0	5 (16.1)	2 (6.5)	4 (12.9)	1 (3.2)	0	0
	Pasta dishes (13)	8 (61.5)	3 (23.1)	6 (46.2)	0	5 (38.5)	0	0	1 (7.7)	0	0
	Pies, unsweetened, or pizzas (18)	11 (61.1)	1 (5.6)	7 (38.9)	0	0	2 (11.1)	4 (2.2)	0	0	0
Miscellaneous food products	Prepared food products (44)	17 (38.6)	4 (9.1)	13 (29.5)	7 (15.9)	6 (13.6)	6 (13.6)	1 (2.3)	0	4 (9.1)	0
	Savory cereal dishes (16)	10 (62.5)	2 (12.5)	1 (6.3)	0	6 (37.5)	6 (37.5)	1 (6.3)	0	0	0
	Savory snacks (28)	7 (25.0)	2 (7.1)	12 (42.9)	7 (25.0)	0	0	0	0	4 (14.3)	0
	Total (629)	200 (31.8)	84 (13.4)	84 (13.4)	83 (13.2)	57 (9.1)	37 (5.9)	23 (3.7)	22 (3.5)	22 (3.5)	20 (3.2)

Results are expressed as frequency (n, number of products including a specific ingredient) and (percentage based on the total products within the category or the subgroup). * Palm fat includes palm kernel or palm stearin. Other fats not included are milk, egg (liquid or powder), or cheese.

Table 4. Sugar addition and types of sugars and sweeteners used in the formulation of gluten free (GF) products.

Food Groups	Food Subgroups (n)	No Added Sugars Declared n (%)	Added Sugar Presence n (%)	Sucrose n (%)	Dextrose n (%)	Other Sugars * n (%)	Glucose and Fructose Syrup n (%)	Non-Refined or Cane Sugar n (%)	Rice Syrup n (%)	Beetroot Sugar Syrup n (%)	Honey n (%)	Lactose n (%)	No-Calorie Sweeteners n (%)
Beverages (non-milk)	Alcoholic beverages (14)	11 (79.0)	3 (21.0)	1 (7.0)	0	2 (14.0)	0	0	0	0	0	0	0
	Beer or beer-like beverages (14)	11 (79.0)	3 (21.0)	1 (7.0)	0	2 (14.0)	0	0	0	0	0	0	0
Milk, milk product, or milk substitutes	Frozen dairy desserts (6)	0	6 (100.0)	6 (100.0)	1 (16.0)	0	5 (83.0)	0	0	0	0	0	0
	Bread and similar (152)	15 (10.0)	137 (90.0)	71 (47.0)	45 (30.0)	3 (2.0)	25 (16.4)	9 (6.0)	23 (15.0)	2 (1.3)	12 (8.0)	0	0
	Bread products (11)	2 (18.0)	9 (82.0)	6 (54.5)	1 (9.0)	0	2 (18.0)	1 (9.0)	0	0	0	0	0
	Leavened breads (89)	2 (2.0)	87 (98.0)	41 (46.0)	28 (31.0)	2 (2.0)	16 (18.0)	7 (8.0)	20 (22.4)	2 (2.0)	12 (13.0)	0	0
	Unleavened breads, crisp breads, and rusks (52)	11 (21.0)	41 (79.0)	24 (46.0)	16 (31.0)	1 (2.0)	7 (13.4)	1 (2.0)	3 (6.0)	0	0	0	0
	Breakfast cereals (40)	8 (20.0)	32 (80.0)	29 (72.5)	3 (7.5)	1 (2.5)	9 (22.5)	4 (10.0)	0	0	3 (7.5)	0	1 (2.5)
	Breakfast cereals (35)	8 (23.0)	27 (77.0)	24 (68.5)	2 (6.0)	0	5 (14.0)	4 (11.4)	0	0	1 (3.0)	0	1 (3.0)
	Cereal bars (5)	0	5 (100.0)	5 (100.0)	1 (20.0)	1 (20.0)	4 (80.0)	0	0	0	2 (40.0)	0	0
Grain or grain products	Cereal or cereal-like milling products and derivatives (25)	11 (44.0)	14 (56.0)	6 (24.0)	7 (28.0)	0	1 (4.0)	3 (12.0)	0	0	0	0	0
	Fine bakery ware (229)	4 (2.1)	225 (98.0)	195 (85.0)	45 (20.0)	7 (3.0)	99 (43.0)	32 (14.0)	6 (3.0)	9 (4.0)	3 (1.3)	4 (2.0)	4 (2.0)
	Biscuits, sweets, and semi-sweets (96)	1 (1.0)	95 (99.0)	74 (77.0)	6 (6.2)	4 (4.1)	34 (35.4)	26 (27.0)	4 (4.1)	9 (9.3)	3 (3.1)	3 (3.1)	3 (3.1)
	Pancakes or waffles (6)	1 (17.0)	5 (83.0)	2 (33.3)	4 (66.6)	0	0	0	0	0	0	0	0
	Pastries and cakes (127)	2 (2.0)	125 (98.0)	119 (94.0)	35 (28.0)	3 (2.3)	65 (51.0)	6 (5.0)	2 (2.0)	0	0	1 (0.7)	1 (0.7)
	Pasta and similar products (88)	87 (99.0)	1 (1.0)	0	0	0	0	1 (1.0)	0	0	0	0	0
	Savory cereal dishes (31)	5 (16.0)	26 (84.0)	10 (32.2)	0	2 (6.4)	7 (22.5)	0	0	0	1 (3.2)	0	0
	Pasta dishes (13)	4 (30.0)	9 (70.0)	6 (46.1)	0	2 (15.3)	5 (38.4)	0	0	0	0	0	0
	Pies, unsweetened, or pizzas (18)	1 (5.5)	17 (94.4)	17 (94.4)	10 (55.5)	0	2 (11.1)	0	0	0	1 (5.5)	0	0
Miscellaneous food products	Prepared food products (44)	13 (30.0)	31 (70.0)	20 (45.4)	4 (9.0)	10 (23)	9 (20.4)	2 (4.5)	2 (4.5)	0	0	2 (4.5)	0
	Savory cereal dishes (16)	1 (6.0)	15 (94.0)	10 (62.5)	3 (19.0)	5 (31.2)	6 (37.5)	0	0	0	0	2 (12.5)	0
	Savory snacks (28)	12 (43.0)	16 (57.0)	10 (36.0)	1 (3.5)	5 (18.0)	3 (11.0)	2 (7.1)	2 (7.1)	0	0	0	0
	Total (629)	154 (24.5)	475 (75.5)	351 (55.8)	115 (18.2)	25 (4.0)	155 (24.6)	51 (8.1)	31 (5.0)	11 (2.0)	19 (3.0)	6 (1.0)	5 (0.7)

Results are expressed as frequency (n, number of products including a specific ingredient) and (percentage based on the total products within the category or the subgroup). * Other sugars include isomaltose, fructose, glucose, agave syrup, golden syrup, maltodextrin, or high maltose corn syrup.

Table 5. Types of fibers used in the formulation of gluten free (GF) products.

Food Groups	Food Subgroups (n)	Xanthan Gum n (%)	Hydroxypropyl Methyl Cellulose n (%)	Guar Gum n (%)	Vegetable Gums * n (%)	Sodium Carboxymethyl Cellulose n (%)	Citrus Fiber n (%)	Carrageenan n (%)	Pectin ** n (%)	Cellulose n (%)	Locust Bean Gum n (%)	Apple Fiber n (%)
Beverages (non-milk)	Alcoholic beverages (14)	0	0	0	0	0	0	0	0	0	0	0
	Beer or beer-like beverages (14)	0	0	0	0	0	0	0	0	0	0	0
Milk, milk product, or milk substitutes	Frozen dairy desserts (6)	0	0	5 (83.3)	0	0	0	1 (16.6)	0	0	2 (33.3)	0
	Bread and similar (152)	77 (50.7)	91 (59.9)	31 (20.4)	75 (49.3)	15 (9.9)	4 (2.6)	0	4 (2.6)	1 (0.7)	0	5 (3.3)
	Bread products (11)	6 (54.5)	4 (36.4)	3 (27.3)	0	0	0	0	0	0	0	0
	Leavened breads (89)	26 (50.0)	25 (48.1)	15 (16.9)	20 (38.5)	1 (1.9)	0	0	0	0	0	0
	Unleavened breads, crisp breads, and rusks (52)	5 (9.6)	9 (17.3)	12 (23.1)	0	0	0	6 (11.5)	1 (1.9)	2 (3.8)	0	4 (7.7)
	Breakfast cereals (40)	0	0	0	2 (5.0)	0	0	0	0	0	0	0
	Breakfast cereals (35)	0	0	0	2 (5.7)	0	0	0	0	0	0	0
	Cereal bars (5)	0	0	0	0	0	0	0	0	0	0	0
Grain or grain products	Cereal or cereal-like milling products and derivatives (25)	4 (16.0)	4 (16.0)	5 (20.0)	1 (4.0)	6 (24.0)	0	2 (8.0)	0	0	0	1 (4.0)
	Fine bakery ware (229)	118 (51.5)	34 (14.8)	51 (22.3)	30 (13.1)	18 (7.9)	12 (5.2)	10 (4.4)	4 (1.7)	7 (3.1)	9 (3.9)	1 (0.4)
	Biscuits, sweets, and semi-sweets (96)	23 (24.0)	1 (1.0)	17 (17.7)	7 (7.3)	0	10 (10.4)	0	0	0	1 (1.0)	0
	Pancakes or waffles (6)	5 (83.3)	0	1 (16.7)	0	1 (16.7)	0	0	0	0	0	0
	Pastries and cakes (127)	90 (70.9)	33 (26.0)	33 (26.0)	23 (18.1)	17 (13.4)	2 (1.6)	10 (7.9)	4 (3.1)	7 (5.5)	8 (6.3)	1 (0.8)
	Pasta and similar products (88)	0	0	1 (1.1)	0	0	0	0	0	0	0	0
	Savory cereal dishes (31)	8 (25.8)	15 (48.8)	21 (67.7)	13 (41.9)	0	0	1 (3.2)	5 (16.1)	5 (16.1)	0	2 (6.5)
	Pasta dishes (13)	3 (23.1)	0	8 (61.5)	6 (46.2)	0	0	0	0	0	0	0
	Pies, unsweetened, or pizzas (18)	5 (27.8)	15 (83.3)	13 (72.2)	7 (38.9)	0	0	1 (5.6)	5 (27.8)	5 (27.8)	0	2 (15.4)
Miscellaneous food products	Prepared food products (44)	8 (18.2)	1 (2.3)	10 (22.7)	2 (4.5)	1 (2.3)	1 (2.3)	0	0	0	1 (2.3)	1 (2.3)
	Savory cereal dishes (16)	8 (50.0)	1 (6.3)	8 (50.0)	2 (12.5)	0	0	0	0	0	1 (6.3)	1 (6.3)
	Savory snacks (28)	0	0	2 (7.1)	0	1 (3.6)	1 (3.6)	0	0	0	0	0
	Total (629)	215 (34.2)	145 (23.1)	124 (19.7)	123 (19.6)	40 (6.4)	17 (2.7)	14 (2.2)	13 (2.1)	13 (2.1)	12 (1.9)	10 (1.6)

Results are expressed as frequency (n, number of products including a specific ingredient) and (percentage based on the total products within the category or the subgroup). * Vegetable gums include psyllium, bamboo, chicory, potato, rice, pea, or corn. ** Extract from apple or other fruits.

Table 6. Energy and nutrient composition per 100 g of gluten free (GF) products, based on the nutritional information on the labels.

Food Groups	Food Subgroups (n)	Energy (kcal)	Fats (Total) (g)	SFA (g)	Carbohydrates (g)	Sugars (g)	Protein (g)	Fiber (g)	Salt (g)
Beverages (non-milk)	Alcoholic beverages (14)	42.4 ± 12.5	0	0	4.2 ± 1.49	1.8 ± 1.5	0.3 ± 0.2	ND	0
	Beer or beer-like beverages (14)	42.4 ± 12.5	0	0	4.2 ± 1.49	1.8 ± 1.5	0.3 ± 0.2	ND	0
Milk, milk product, or milk substitutes	Frozen dairy desserts (6)	291.8 ± 115.6	12.5 ± 4.7	8.8 ± 4.2	33.1 ± 10.4	21.4 ± 3.7	3.3 ± 1.1	1.7 ± 0.7	0.1 ± 0.0
	Bread and similar (152)	318.3 ± 69.4	6.8 ± 5.8	2.5 ± 3.1	58.7 ± 15.5	4.3 ± 3.2	3.1 ± 2.1	5.2 ± 2.2	1.5 ± 0.5
	Bread products (11)	369.0 ± 28.8	3.3 ± 3.6	1.1 ± 1.6	78.5 ± 7.1	2.8 ± 2.7	4.1 ± 2.1	3.1 ± 2.0	1.5 ± 0.5
	Leavened breads (89)	283.9 ± 50.7	5.7 ± 3.3	2.2 ± 2.6	52.4 ± 11.7	5.2 ± 3.4	2.7 ± 1.6	5.8 ± 1.9	1.4 ± 0.4
	Unleavened breads, crisp breads, and rusks (52)	366.5 ± 68.3	9.3 ± 8.2	3.2 ± 3.9	65.2 ± 16.6	3.0 ± 2.2	3.6 ± 2.6	4.5 ± 2.4	1.7 ± 0.6
	Breakfast cereals (40)	381.3 ± 35.9	5.4 ± 4.9	1.7 ± 1.8	73.0 ± 12.8	17.0 ± 11.4	7.5 ± 2.6	5.2 ± 3.4	0.6 ± 0.6
	Breakfast cereals (35)	385.0 ± 26.4	4.5 ± 4.5	1.3 ± 1.4	75.6 ± 9.2	15.4 ± 10.8	7.9 ± 2.5	5.2 ± 3.4	0.6 ± 0.6
	Cereal bars (5)	355.0 ± 75.3	12.2 ± 1.6	4.5 ± 1.8	54.9 ± 20.2	27.6 ± 10.2	5.1 ± 1.7	4.9 ± 3.9	0.2 ± 0.2
Grain or grain products	Cereal or cereal-like milling products and derivatives (25)	337.1 ± 39.7	2.1 ± 2.5	0.7 ± 1.3	73.0 ± 13.1	8.1 ± 10.8	3.9 ± 2.6	4.5 ± 3.4	0.6 ± 0.7
	Fine bakery ware (229)	426.1 ± 77.6	20.5 ± 6.8	8.1 ± 5.4	55.3 ± 12.1	22.2 ± 9.2	4.1 ± 1.6	3.2 ± 2.1	0.7 ± 0.5
	Biscuits, sweets, and semi-sweets (96)	471.5 ± 41.8	19.9 ± 5.9	9.4 ± 5.5	67.5 ± 6.4	25.5 ± 8.3	4.4 ± 1.4	3.5 ± 2.3	0.6 ± 0.5
	Pancakes or waffles (6)	237.9 ± 122.2	9.3 ± 8.7	3.4 ± 4.2	36.5 ± 11.1	6.5 ± 10.9	1.7 ± 1.5	ND	0.8 ± 0.1
	Pastries and cakes (127)	400.6 ± 71.4	21.4 ± 6.8	7.3 ± 5.1	47.0 ± 8.1	20.5 ± 8.6	4.0 ± 1.7	3.0 ± 1.7	0.8 ± 0.6
	Pasta and similar products (88)	347.3 ± 25.5	1.3 ± 0.7	0.2 ± 0.3	76.5 ± 5.9	1.0 ± 0.5	6.4 ± 1.2	2.2 ± 1.7	0.04 ± 0.1
	Savory cereal dishes (31)	224.5 ± 55.5	7.9 ± 2.9	3.5 ± 1.6	29.7 ± 15.2	2.4 ± 1.8	7.7 ± 2.0	2.7 ± 1.7	1.1 ± 0.5
	Pasta dishes (13)	216.0 ± 82.1	6.6 ± 3.4	2.9 ± 1.8	31.5 ± 23.1	2.9 ± 2.6	6.8 ± 2.0	2.3 ± 1.9	0.9 ± 0.6
	Pies, unsweetened, or pizzas (18)	230.6 ± 24.3	8.8 ± 2.0	4.0 ± 1.2	28.4 ± 5.3	2.1 ± 0.8	8.4 ± 1.8	3.0 ± 1.4	1.3 ± 0.4
Miscellaneous food products	Prepared food products (44)	351.1 ± 132.8	9.9 ± 7.5	4.1 ± 4.5	58.7 ± 25.0	6.5 ± 10.3	5.6 ± 2.2	2.4 ± 1.4	1.2 ± 0.7
	Savory cereal dishes (16)	196.9 ± 87.0	6.2 ± 4.9	2.1 ± 2.2	30.1 ± 18.1	1.9 ± 1.8	4.7 ± 2.1	1.4 ± 0.9	1.1 ± 0.5
	Savory snacks (28)	439.1 ± 42.1	12.0 ± 7.9	5.2 ± 5.1	75.1 ± 7.3	9.0 ± 12.1	6.1 ± 2.1	2.8 ± 1.3	1.2 ± 0.8
Total (629)		302.2 ± 62.7	7.4 ± 4.0	3.3 ± 2.5	51.4 ± 12.5	9.4 ± 5.8	4.7 ± 1.7	3.4 ± 2.1	0.6 ± 0.4

Data are expressed as average ± standard deviation. SFA, saturated fatty acids.

Many of the considered GF food products showed very high contents of: energy (33.5%), defined as >400 kcal/100 g; fats (28.4%), defined as >17.5 g/100 g; saturated fatty acids (30.0%), defined as >5 g/100 g; sugars (21.6%), defined as >22.5 g/100 g; and salt (28.3%), defined as >500 mg of sodium or the equivalent value for salt /100 g. On the other hand, 25.4% could be labeled as a source of fiber (>3 g/100 g) [21,22].

4. Discussion

This cross-sectional study of 629 cereal-based GF products represents the largest comparative nutrient analysis of packaged Spanish GF food products and their ingredients, up to date. Most of the considered GF food products (~ 30%) showed very high contents of energy, fats, saturated fatty acids, sugars, and salt. In contrast, 25.4% could be labeled as a source of fiber [21,22]. Compared to other recent studies, our food composition database showed similar or slightly lower nutrient values than others [23–27].

It is important to mention that there is not an unequivocal nutritional profile for GF food products worldwide. Differences from country to country, from brand to brand, and among food categories have been asserted. Furthermore, differences could be attributable to different methodology (product selection) between studies. Nutritional values of each food item included in the present database were calculated as average of all the single similar foods from each brand included in each category. Therefore, nutritional composition variability for each food item due to its ingredient formulation has been considered.

Regarding ingredients, we found that the main fat component of GF products was sunflower oil, followed by palm fat, olive oil, and cocoa fat. This result differs to that shown by Calvo-Lerma et al. [25] in a similar study conducted in Spain, in which they found that GF products were largely composed of palm oil. Our database was developed up to March 2019 and the data collection in the study by Calvo-Lerma et al. [25] was conducted between March and October 2017. In this sense, this could indicate recent food reformulation to improve the nutritional quality of fat, thus providing a healthier food choice for celiac patients. In fact, recent research on palm fat and oil has brought up intriguing health issues, due to the presence of toxic contaminants generated in the processing of palm oil and other vegetable oils. This has promoted an update on the tolerable daily intakes (TDI) for toxic contaminants (2- and 3-monochloropropanediols and glycidyl esters [28,29]), but has also posed some misunderstandings in mass communication [28]. Consumers have been aware of these issues through the media, demanding and purchasing only palm oil free biscuits, especially for children. Processed foods are constantly changing as manufacturers try to protect or increase market share and profits and respond to policy changes dictated by a combination of government policies and consumer pressure, e.g., reduction of sugar, salt, saturated, and trans fatty acids [30]. General awareness of the role of diet on health is boosting the rate of changes in composition and foods consumed in many countries.

In the case of breads, we found that fat was commonly added to leavened breads, being it sunflower oil in more than 50% of the cases, followed by olive oil and a margarine made with palm, coconut, and sunflower oils. Consequent nutritional composition renders a considerably high amount of fat (5.7 %), most of it unsaturated (61%). Our data are slightly lower than those given by Calvo Lerma et al. [25] for total fat in a study of 619 GF products conducted in 2017. Miranda et al. [10] also studied Spanish GF commercialized breads in a study of 206 GF products, undertaken between 2012 and 2013, and stated that these contained less protein and double the fat content, (being this fat mainly SFA), in contrast to their gluten containing counterparts. Again, producers may be reducing fat in leavened breads, although data show that there is a large variability in fat composition when comparing different brands.

Fat content in pastries, cakes, pancakes, or waffles was 30% saturated and the most commonly added fat was palm fat. Results are in agreement with other studies [10,25].

GF products are made with high amounts of fat and sugar to achieve a texture resembling the typical and unique wheat viscoelastic properties [18,19]. Fat ingredients are indeed useful in bakery products for the stabilization of gas bubbles and the reduction of kneading resistance and swelling of starch granules [31]. Moreover, emulsifiers can be used to increase dough stiffness, improve bread structure, and decrease the speed of staling. In pasta products, emulsifiers act as lubricants in the extrusion process and provide firmer consistency and a less sticky surface, as they control starch swelling and leaching phenomena during cooking [32]. Other components such as sugars (sucrose, glucose, and fructose syrup), starch (corn starch, rice flour, and corn flour), and fibers (xanthan gum, hydroxypropyl methyl cellulose, and guar gum) were also present in GF products in our database.

It is interesting to point out that almost all breads contained added sugars (98% of leavened breads and 79% of unleavened breads, crisps, and rusks). Sugar is not a common ingredient in bread. In Spain, normal bread is solely composed of flour (usually wheat), salt, baker's yeast, and water [33], although sugar may be added to special breads. Sugar addition in bread is normally a matter of concern since bread is not usually associated with sugar consumption in the population. Due to the sugar addition, simple carbohydrate composition raised to values around 5.2 g per 100 g. This amount is similar to that described by Miranda et al. [10] in 2012–2013, and somewhat smaller than that described by Calvo Lerma et al. [25] in 2017. Nonetheless, both authors state that there is no significant difference in sugar content when comparing GF breads with their gluten containing counterparts. Therefore, gluten-containing flour may be contributing to sugar composition on a higher amount as compared to GF flour. To prove this idea, sugar content in GF pasta, without added sugars, was quite low (below 1%), and other authors have demonstrated that GF pasta contains a significantly lower amount of sugars as compared to gluten containing pasta [10,25].

Cereal-based GF products were primarily composed of rice and/or corn flour. Less than 10% of the GF products were formulated with other kind of flours, such as buckwheat, soy and other legumes, brown rice, millet, or quinoa. Therefore, the type of flour used results in a high glycemic index, because of the high content (70–80%) of amylopectin and related glucose polymers. The use of pseudocereals is still small, although several authors present them as good gluten free alternatives. According to Jastrebova and Jägerstad [34], the best way to develop nutritious healthy GF products with high content of proteins, fibers, micronutrients, and antioxidants, is natural fortification by using nutritious ingredients such as whole grain flours of GF cereals/pseudocereals, protein-rich flours of soy, lupin, chick-pea, chestnut, and different seeds, as well as bioprocessing, such as germination or fermentation with yeast and/or sourdough. Other authors suggest the use of pseudocereals such as amaranth, quinoa, or buckwheat because of their content in thiamine, vitamin E, or carotenoids [35] or the nutritional quality of their protein, fat, fiber, and minerals [36].

In our study, soy, legume, and quinoa flours were present in 8.4%, 7.3% and 4.1%, respectively, of the analyzed products. Breakfast cereals were the group with the most frequent inclusion of alternative cereals such as teff, oatmeal, sorghum, and other flours coming from chia, amaranth, or flaxseeds. Again, manufacturers seem to be timidly introducing the use of nutritious pseudocereal and legume flours in the formulation of GF products.

Xanthan gum and hydroxypropyl methylcellulose are the most popular hydrocolloids that are used in GF products. They display thickening properties through the binding of water and, as a result, the viscosity of the gluten-free dough is enhanced and gas is better retained, improving loaf volume and structure [14].

Differences between GF products and their equivalents with gluten have also been described in other studies. The most recent surveys on the nutritional quality of GF food products currently available on the market, and recently reviewed by Melini and Melini [18], show key inadequacies—a low protein content and a high fat and salt content—compared to their equivalent gluten-containing products. However, an interesting trend towards some improvements has emerged. More adequate levels of fiber and sugar than in the past have been reported in the surveys of the last two years, although the composition in terms of fiber and sugars is highly variable between the different product categories. Further studies are nevertheless required to investigate the micronutrient content of GF food products, since very few reported data exist. Kulai and Rashid [37] and Jamieson et al. [26]

informed of a significant lower iron and folate content in GF products compared to gluten containing food. Potassium content was also significantly lower in GF food products [27]. Furthermore, only 5% of GF breads were fortified with all four mandatory fortification nutrients (calcium, iron, nicotinic acid or nicotinamide, and thiamin), and 28% of GF breads were fortified with calcium and iron only in UK [24]. Fortified GF products represent only 10% of GF staple foods in Europe, because the use of starches (with low levels of many essential micronutrients) as main ingredient in many GF foods makes it difficult to implement common fortification with single micronutrients [34]. This lack of fortification may increase the risk of micronutrient deficiency in coeliac sufferers according to these authors. GF choices could account in unanticipated health disorders for CD patients based on the limited labeling description and narrow range of nutritionally balanced products and brands currently available [25].

Average salt content in all products was 0.6 g/100 g. As compared to other studies [10], we found much lower amounts of salt in pasta, cereal milling products, and fine bakery ware. Other studies [25] do not show data on salt content since salt content in nutritional information labels was only introduced as compulsory from December 2016 [38]. As with fat quality, salt reduction could be another of the reformulation targets that are being assessed in GF products.

Several population studies, in different countries, have investigated the nutritional status of CD patients adhering to a GFD. In published studies, CD patients consumed more fats (especially saturated), protein, and simple carbohydrates (sugars) but less fiber and micronutrients, such as iron, calcium, and vitamin D than recommended [11,17,39,40], and also compared to healthy subjects [16,41,42]. A research group from our laboratory recently showed no relevant differences in the general nutrient quality of the diet of children and adolescents following a GFD, as compared to matched controls, in contrast to previous studies, with the exception of polyunsaturated fatty acids, folate, and calcium intakes. These were significantly lower in coeliac as compared to non-coeliac children and adolescents, as well as low when compared to the recommended intakes for these nutrients [13]. Adequacy of vitamin D intake to recommendations was dramatically low, for both coeliac and non-coeliac children and adolescents; however, only coeliac girls presented a significantly lower level of plasmatic vitamin D (below reference values, <30 ng/mL), as compared to non-coeliac controls, although without clinical repercussion in bone mass density [13]. Therefore, we consider that vitamin D fortification in GF products could be a strategy of great importance to minimize adverse health effects associated to vitamin D deficiency.

5. Conclusions

In conclusion, the present study represents an attempt to build a systematic composition database of GF products based on the ingredients listed on the label and the nutritional information provided by the manufacturer. This type of study is a priority, since CD patients include this type of products in their diets, and studies assessing CD patient's diets need to use updated data on GF product composition. Moreover, since nutritional deficiencies have been described for CD patients and it has been shown that nutritional quality of GF products is lower, updated quality assessment of available products is needed for further improvement in GF product development. We describe 629 cereal-based GF products available in the Spanish market, in terms of ingredients and strategic nutrients. However, information on micronutrient composition is a still pending question.

5.1. Strengths

Studies that evaluate the formulations of commercially available GF products are scarce. In our study, we included an important number (629) of products and we describe them using a standardized classification (LanguaL™ Thesaurus EuroFIR), in order to make them comparable to other studies. Brands have also been recorded. Our data are likely to be just as accurate as most data reported for any kind of food product present on the market.

5.2. Limitations

Some limitations related to our data should be considered. First, since the nutritional composition data of GF products has been estimated, it cannot substitute a direct analysis. Direct chemical analysis is the gold standard to estimate the nutrient composition of food. Additionally, nutrient data shown on food labels provided by the food industry may be based on estimations from the ingredients rather than direct chemical analysis of the food products. Finally, another limitation is related to the lack of information on micronutrient content (minerals and vitamins) in GF products.

Author Contributions: E.A.-A. and N.Ú. designed, wrote the manuscript, supervised, and carried out the project administration. E.A.-A. and N.Ú., and V.F. were responsible for interpretation and discussion of the results. V.F., M.P.G., and M.d.L.S.-V. contributed to the review of the study protocol, design, and methodology. V.F., M.P.G., M.d.L.S.-V. and M.M. were responsible for the careful software, resources, formal analysis, and investigation. V.F., and M.P.G. designed, wrote—reviewed and edited the manuscript. E.A.-A., N.Ú., and M.A. revised the manuscript, and shared funding acquisition. E.A.-A., the Principal Investigator, was responsible for the design, protocol, methodology, and follow-up/checking of the study. All authors have read and agreed to the published version of the manuscript.

Funding: This study was supported by a Grant FUSPBS-PPC08-2015 from Universidad CEU San Pablo, Madrid (Spain).

Conflicts of Interest: The authors declare no conflict of interest.

References

1. Singh, P.; Arora, A.; Strand, T.A.; Leffler, D.A.; Catassi, C.; Green, P.H.; Kelly, C.P.; Ahuja, V.; Makharia, G.K. Global prevalence of celiac disease: Systematic review and meta-analysis. *Clin. Gastroenterol. Hepatol.* **2018**, *16*, 823–836. [CrossRef] [PubMed]
2. Leonard, M.M.; Sapone, A.; Catassi, C.; Fasano, A. Celiac disease and nonceliac gluten sensitivity: A review. *Jama* **2017**, *318*, 647–656. [CrossRef] [PubMed]
3. Bascuñán, K.A.; Vespa, M.C.; Araya, M. Celiac disease: Understanding the gluten-free diet. *Eur. J. Nutr.* **2017**, *56*, 449–459. [CrossRef] [PubMed]
4. Gobbetti, M.; Pontonio, E.; Filannino, P.; Rizzello, C.G.; De Angelis, M.; Di Cagno, R. How to improve the gluten-free diet: The state of the art from a food science perspective. *Food Res. Int.* **2018**, *110*, 22–32. [CrossRef] [PubMed]
5. Comission Implementing Regulation (EU) No 828/2014 of 30 July 2014 on the requirements for the provision of information to consumers on the absence or reduced presence of gluten in food Text with EEA relevance. *Off. J. Eur. Union* **2014**, *L228*, 5–8. Available online: https://eur-lex.europa.eu/eli/reg_impl/2014/828/oj (accessed on 21 October 2019).
6. Rai, S.; Kaur, A.; Chopra, C.S. Gluten-free products for celiac susceptible people. *Front. Nutr.* **2018**, *5*, 116. [CrossRef]
7. Verrill, L.; Zhang, Y.; Kane, R. Food label usage and reported difficulty with following a gluten-free diet among individuals in the USA with coeliac disease and those with nonceliac gluten sensitivity. *J. Hum. Nutr. Diet.* **2013**, *26*, 479–487. [CrossRef]
8. Fiormarkets. Gluten-Free Products Market by Types (Pasta and Rice, Prepared Foods, Desserts & Ice Creams, Condiments, Seasonings, Spreads, Meats/Meats Alternatives, Dairy/Dairy Alternatives, Bakery Products), Distribution Channel (Drug Stores, Club Stores, Health Food Store, Mass Merchandiser, Grocery Stores), Region, Global Industry Analysis, Market Size, Share, Growth, Trends, and Forecast 2020 to 2027. 2020. Available online: https://www.fiormarkets.com/report/gluten-free-products-market-by-types-pasta-and-rice-418071.html (accessed on 15 June 2020).
9. Hartmann, C.; Hieke, S.; Taper, C.; Siegrist, M. European consumer healthiness evaluation of 'free-from' labelled food products. *Food Qual. Prefer.* **2018**, *68*, 377–388. [CrossRef]
10. Miranda, J.; Lasa, A.; Bustamante, M.; Churruca, I.; Simon, E. Nutritional differences between a gluten-free diet and a diet containing equivalent products with gluten. *Plant Food Hum. Nutr.* **2014**, *69*, 182–187. [CrossRef]
11. Rybicka, I. The Handbook of minerals on a gluten-free diet. *Nutrients* **2018**, *10*, 1683. [CrossRef]

12. Larretxi, I.; Txurruka, I.; Navarro, V.; Lasa, A.; Bustamante, M.A.; Fernandez-Gil, M.D.; Simon, E.; Miranda, J. Micronutrient analysis of gluten-free products: Their low content is not involved in gluten-free diet imbalance in a cohort of celiac children and adolescent. *Foods* **2019**, *8*, 321. [CrossRef] [PubMed]
13. Ballestero, C.; Varela-Moreiras, G.; Úbeda, N.; Alonso-Aperte, E. Nutritional status in Spanish children and adolescents with celiac disease on a gluten free diet compared to non-celiac disease controls. *Nutrients* **2019**, *11*, 2329. [CrossRef] [PubMed]
14. El Khoury, D.; Balfour-Ducharme, S.; Joye, I.J. A review on the gluten-free diet: Technological and nutritional challenges. *Nutrients* **2018**, *10*, 1410. [CrossRef] [PubMed]
15. Larretxi, I.; Simon, E.; Benjumea, L.; Miranda, J.; Bustamante, M.A.; Lasa, A.; Eizaguirre, F.J.; Churruca, I. Gluten-free-rendered products contribute to imbalanced diets in children and adolescents with celiac disease. *Eur. J. Nutr.* **2019**, *58*, 775–783. [CrossRef] [PubMed]
16. Barone, M.; Della Valle, N.; Rosania, R.; Facciorusso, A.; Trotta, A.; Cantatore, F.P.; Falco, S.; Pignatiello, S.; Viggiani, M.T.; Amoruso, A.; et al. A comparison of the nutritional status between adult celiac patients on a long-term, strictly gluten-free diet and healthy subjects. *Eur. J. Clin. Nutr.* **2016**, *70*, 23–27. [CrossRef] [PubMed]
17. Shepherd, S.; Gibson, P. Nutritional inadequacies of the gluten-free diet in both recently-diagnosed and long-term patients with coeliac disease. *J. Hum. Nutr. Diet.* **2013**, *26*, 349–358. [CrossRef]
18. Melini, V.; Melini, F. Gluten-free diet: Gaps and needs for a healthier diet. *Nutrients* **2019**, *11*, 170. [CrossRef]
19. Taetzsch, A.; Das, S.K.; Brown, C.; Krauss, A.; Silver, R.E.; Roberts, S.B. Are gluten-free diets more nutritious? An evaluation of self-selected and recommended gluten-free and gluten-containing dietary patterns. *Nutrients* **2018**, *10*, 1881. [CrossRef]
20. Møller, A.; Ireland, J. LanguaL™ 2017—The LanguaL™ Thesaurus. Technical Report. *Danish Food Inf.* **2018**. [CrossRef]
21. Comission Regulation (EC) No 1924/2006 of the European Parliament and of the Council of 20 December 2006 on nutrition and health claims made on foods. *Off. J. Eur. Union* **2006**, *L404*, 9–25. Available online: https://eur-lex.europa.eu/legal-content/en/ALL/?uri=CELEX%3A32006R1924 (accessed on 22 January 2020).
22. Food Standards Agency. *Guide to Creating a Front of Pack (fop) Nutrition Label for Pre-Packed Products Sold Through Retail Outlets*; Department of Health: London, UK, 2016; p. 33. Available online: https://www.gov.uk/government/publications (accessed on 27 January 2020).
23. Fry, L.; Madden, A.; Fallaize, R. An investigation into the nutritional composition and cost of gluten-free versus regular food products in the UK. *J. Hum. Nutr. Diet.* **2018**, *31*, 108–120. [CrossRef] [PubMed]
24. Allen, B.; Orfila, C. The availability and nutritional adequacy of gluten-free bread and pasta. *Nutrients* **2018**, *10*, 1370. [CrossRef] [PubMed]
25. Calvo-Lerma, J.; Crespo-Escobar, P.; Martinez-Barona, S.; Fornes-Ferrer, V.; Donat, E.; Ribes-Koninckx, C. Differences in the macronutrient and dietary fibre profile of gluten-free products as compared to their gluten-containing counterparts. *Eur. J. Clin. Nutr.* **2019**, *73*, 930–936. [CrossRef] [PubMed]
26. Jamieson, J.A.; Weir, M.; Gougeon, L. Canadian packaged gluten-free foods are less nutritious than their regular gluten-containing counterparts. *PeerJ* **2018**, *6*, e5875. [CrossRef]
27. Missbach, B.; Schwingshackl, L.; Billmann, A.; Mystek, A.; Hickelsberger, M.; Bauer, G.; König, J. Gluten-free food database: The nutritional quality and cost of packaged gluten-free foods. *PeerJ* **2015**, *3*, e1337. [CrossRef]
28. Gesteiro, E.; Guijarro, L.; Sánchez-Muniz, F.J.; Vidal-Carou, M.d.C.; Troncoso, A.; Venanci, L.; Jimeno, V.; Quilez, J.; Anadón, A.; González-Gross, M. Palm oil on the edge. *Nutrients* **2019**, *11*, 2008. [CrossRef]
29. EFSA Panel on Contaminants in the Food Chain (CONTAM). Update of the risk assessment on 3-monochloropropane diol and its fatty acid esters. *EFSA J.* **2018**, *16*, 508. [CrossRef]
30. Kapsokefalou, M.; Roe, M.; Turrini, A.; Costa, H.S.; Martinez-Victoria, E.; Marletta, L.; Berry, R.; Finglas, P. Food composition at present: New challenges. *Nutrients* **2019**, *11*, 1714. [CrossRef]
31. Houben, A.; Höchstötter, A.; Becker, T. Possibilities to increase the quality in gluten-free bread production: An overview. *Eur. Food Res. Technol.* **2012**, *235*, 195–208. [CrossRef]
32. Marti, A.; Pagani, M.A. What can play the role of gluten in gluten free pasta? *Trends Food Sci. Technol.* **2013**, *31*, 63–71. [CrossRef]
33. Real Decreto 308/2019, de 26 de abril, por el que se aprueba la norma de calidad para el pan. *BOE*. **2019**, pp. 50168–50175. Available online: https://www.boe.es/eli/es/rd/2019/04/26/308 (accessed on 26 February 2020).

34. Jastrebova, J.; Jägerstad, M. Novel fortification strategies for staple gluten-free products. In *Handbook of Food Fortification and Health: From Concepts to Public Health Applications*; Preedy, V.R., Srirajaskanthan, R., Patel, V., Eds.; Springer Science+Business Media: New York, NY, USA, 2013; Volume 1, pp. 307–320. [CrossRef]
35. Niro, S.; D'Agostino, A.; Fratianni, A.; Cinquanta, L.; Panfili, G. Gluten-free alternative grains: Nutritional evaluation and bioactive compounds. *Foods* **2019**, *8*, 208. [CrossRef] [PubMed]
36. Martinez-Villaluenga, C.; Penas, E.; Hernandez-Ledesma, B. Pseudocereal grains: Nutritional value, health benefits and current applications for the development of gluten-free foods. *Food Chem. Toxicol.* **2020**, *137*. [CrossRef] [PubMed]
37. Kulai, T.; Rashid, M. Assessment of nutritional adequacy of packaged gluten-free food products. *Can. J. Diet Pract. Res.* **2014**, *75*, 186–190. [CrossRef] [PubMed]
38. Comission Regulation (EU) No 1169/2011 of the European Parliament and of the Council of 25 October 2011 on the provision of food information to consumers, amending Regulations (EC) No 1924/2006 and (EC) No 1925/2006 of the European Parliament and of the Council, and repealing Commission Directive 87/250/EEC, Council Directive 90/496/EEC, Commission Directive 1999/10/EC, Directive 2000/13/EC of the European Parliament and of the Council, Commission Directives 2002/67/EC and 2008/5/EC and Commission Regulation (EC) No 608/2004 (Text with EEA relevance). *Off. J. Eur. Union* **2011**, *L304*, 18–63. Available online: https://eur-lex.europa.eu/legal-content/EN/ALL/?uri=CELEX%3A32011R1169 (accessed on 23 March 2020).
39. Nestares, T.; Martín-Masot, R.; Labella, A.; Aparicio, V.A.; Flor-Alemany, M.; López-Frías, M.; Maldonado, J. Is a gluten-free diet enough to maintain correct micronutrients status in young patients with celiac disease? *Nutrients* **2020**, *12*, 844. [CrossRef] [PubMed]
40. Salazar Quero, J.C.; Espín Jaime, B.; Rodríguez Martínez, A.; Argüelles Martín, F.; García Jiménez, R.; Rubio Murillo, M.; Pizarro Martín, A. Nutritional assessment of gluten-free diet. Is gluten-free diet deficient in some nutrient? *An. Pediatr. (Barc.)* **2015**, *83*, 33–39. [CrossRef]
41. Babio, N.; Alcazar, M.; Castillejo, G.; Recasens, M.; Martinez-Cerezo, F.; Gutierrez-Pensado, V.; Masip, G.; Vaque, C.; Vila-Marti, A.; Torres-Moreno, M.; et al. Patients with celiac disease reported higher consumption of added sugar and total fat than healthy individuals. *J. Pediatr. Gastroenterol. Nutr.* **2017**, *64*, 63–69. [CrossRef]
42. Zuccotti, G.; Fabiano, V.; Dilillo, D.; Picca, M.; Cravidi, C.; Brambilla, P. Intakes of nutrients in Italian children with celiac disease and the role of commercially available gluten-free products. *J. Hum. Nutr. Diet.* **2013**, *26*, 436–444. [CrossRef]

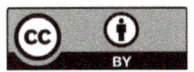

© 2020 by the authors. Licensee MDPI, Basel, Switzerland. This article is an open access article distributed under the terms and conditions of the Creative Commons Attribution (CC BY) license (http://creativecommons.org/licenses/by/4.0/).

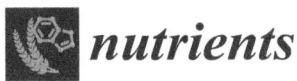

Article

Beneficial Effects of a Low-Nickel Diet on Relapsing IBS-Like and Extraintestinal Symptoms of Celiac Patients during a Proper Gluten-Free Diet: Nickel Allergic Contact Mucositis in Suspected Non-Responsive Celiac Disease

Raffaele Borghini [1], Natascia De Amicis [1], Antonino Bella [2], Nicoletta Greco [1], Giuseppe Donato [1] and Antonio Picarelli [1,*]

[1] Department of Translational and Precision Medicine, Sapienza University, 00185 Rome, Italy; raffaele.borghini@uniroma1.it (R.B.); n.deamicis@libero.it (N.D.A.); nicoletta.greco25@gmail.com (N.G.); giuseppe.donato@uniroma1.it (G.D.)
[2] Department of Infectious Diseases, Istituto Superiore di Sanità, 00161 Rome, Italy; antonio.bella@iss.it
* Correspondence: antonio.picarelli@uniroma1.it

Received: 29 June 2020; Accepted: 24 July 2020; Published: 29 July 2020

Abstract: Background and Aim: Nickel (Ni)-rich foods can induce allergic contact mucositis (ACM) with irritable bowel syndrome (IBS)-like symptoms in predisposed subjects. Ni ACM has a high prevalence (>30%) in the general population and can be diagnosed by a Ni oral mucosa patch test (omPT). Many celiac disease (CD) patients on a gluten-free diet (GFD) often show a recrudescence of gastrointestinal and extraintestinal symptoms, although serological and histological remission has been achieved. Since a GFD often results in higher loads of ingested alimentary Ni (e.g., corn), we hypothesized that it would lead to a consequent intestinal sensitization to Ni in predisposed subjects. We wanted to (1) study Ni ACM prevalence in still symptomatic CD patients on a GFD and (2) study the effects of a low-Ni diet (LNiD) on their recurrent symptoms. Material and Methods: We recruited 102 consecutive CD patients (74 female, 28 male; age range 18–65 years, mean age 42.3 ± 7.4) on a GFD since at least 12 months, in current serological and histological remission (Marsh–Oberhuber type 0–I) who complained of relapsing gastrointestinal and/or extraintestinal symptoms. Inclusion criteria: presence of at least three gastrointestinal symptoms with a score ≥5 on the modified Gastrointestinal Symptom Rating Scale (GSRS) questionnaire. Exclusion criteria: IgE-mediated food allergy; history of past or current cancer; inflammatory bowel diseases; infectious diseases including *Helicobacter pylori*; lactose intolerance. All patients enrolled underwent Ni omPT and followed a LNiD for 3 months. A 24 symptoms questionnaire (GSRS modified according to the Salerno Experts' Criteria, with 15 gastrointestinal and 9 extraintestinal symptoms) was administered at T0 (free diet), T1 (GFD, CD remission), T2 (recurrence of symptoms despite GFD), and T3 (GFD + LNiD) for comparisons. Comparisons were performed using Wilcoxon signed-rank test. RESULTS: Twenty patients (all female, age range 23–65 years, mean age 39.1 ± 2.9) out of 102 (19.6%) were finally included. All 20 patients enrolled (100%) showed positive Ni omPT, confirming an Ni ACM diagnosis. A correct GFD (T0 vs. T1) induced the improvement of 19 out of the total 24 (79.2%) symptoms, and 14 out of 24 (58.3%) were statistically significant (p-value <0.0083 according to Bonferroni correction). Prolonged GFD (T1 vs. T2) revealed the worsening of 20 out of the total 24 (83.3%) symptoms, and 10 out of 24 (41.7%) were statistically significant. LNiD (T2 vs. T3) determined an improvement of 20 out of the total 24 (83.4%) symptoms, and in 10 out of 24 (41.7%) symptoms the improvement was statistically significant. Conclusions: Our data suggest that the recrudescence of gastrointestinal and extraintestinal symptoms observed in CD subjects during GFD may be due to the increase in alimentary Ni intake, once gluten contamination and persisting villous atrophy are excluded. Ni overload can induce Ni ACM, which can be diagnosed by a specific Ni omPT. Improvement of symptoms occurs after a proper LNiD. These encouraging data should be confirmed with larger studies.

Keywords: celiac disease; refractory celiac disease; remission; gluten-free diet; nickel allergy; allergic contact mucositis; irritable bowel syndrome (IBS); low-nickel diet

1. Introduction

Celiac disease (CD) is a chronic inflammatory bowel disease triggered by the ingestion of gluten in genetically susceptible individuals, who test positive for human leukocyte antigen (HLA) DQ2 and/or DQ8. Its prevalence is about 1%, and since the small intestine is its main target organ, CD can have gluten-related gastrointestinal manifestations, such as bloating, abdominal pain, diarrhea, and constipation [1–3]. What is more, CD is a multisystem disorder, and patients can also complain of extraintestinal signs and symptoms [4,5]. CD diagnosis in adults is usually based on positive results of specific serological tests for anti-endomysial antibodies (EMA) and anti-tissue transglutaminase (tTG) antibodies performed during a free diet and then confirmed by the finding of intestinal villous atrophy on histological examination of duodenal biopsies. The only treatment currently available is a lifelong and strict gluten-free diet (GFD) but, nevertheless, many CD patients complain about the persistence or relapse of symptoms even during GFD [6]: in this case, interviews with gastroenterologists and nutritionists are necessary in order to investigate a proper adherence to the GFD; moreover, repetition of serological tests and duodenal biopsies are mandatory to exclude ongoing intestinal damage and gluten exposure. When persistent damage in the duodenal mucosa is found despite a correct GFD, refractory CD and possible complications such as intestinal lymphoma must be investigated [7].

Moreover, in clinically non-responding CD, other possible overlapping diagnoses should be considered, such as inflammatory bowel diseases (IBD), and irritable bowel syndrome (IBS)-like disorders (e.g., lactose intolerance), but many cases seem to remain unsolved [8]. Recently, a diet low in fermentable oligo-, di-, and monosaccharides and polyols (FODMAPs) has been proposed as an ex adiuvantibus treatment to reduce IBS-like symptoms in CD patients following a GFD, although there is no specific indication or supporting diagnostic test [9,10].

More recently, nickel (Ni) allergic contact mucositis (ACM), which is linked to the ingestion of Ni-rich foods, has been added to IBS-like disorders. Together with Ni allergic contact dermatitis (ACD), Ni ACM is an expression of "systemic Ni allergy syndrome" (SNAS) and can have both gastrointestinal and extraintestinal manifestations. According to the European Surveillance System on Contact Allergy (ESSCA), the prevalence of an epicutaneous patch test positive to Ni may reach 30% in some European countries, but Ni ACM prevalence may even be higher [11]. Patients affected by Ni ACM show a low-grade intestinal inflammation with a local adaptive response to Ni-containing foods: this mucositis seems to be characterized by increased lymphocyte trafficking (type IV immune response) [12,13]. Ni ACM diagnosis is currently based on a Ni oral mucosa patch test (omPT), which has already proved good sensitivity and specificity [13], and a low-Ni diet (LNiD) can be thus suggested in this condition in order to significantly reduce both Ni-related gastrointestinal and extraintestinal symptoms [14–19].

Figure 1 shows the main foods with the highest Ni content, and it is easy to observe that many of them (e.g., corn) are consumed in large quantities by CD patients on a proper and strict GFD [15,16]. It is therefore possible that a high load of alimentary Ni may induce or exacerbate a "Ni sensitivity" in predisposed subjects, especially in CD patients on a long-term GFD.

On these premises, our aims were (1) to study the prevalence of Ni ACM in CD patients in serological and histological remission with relapsing symptoms; (2) to evaluate the effects of an LNiD on gastrointestinal and extraintestinal symptoms in these patients.

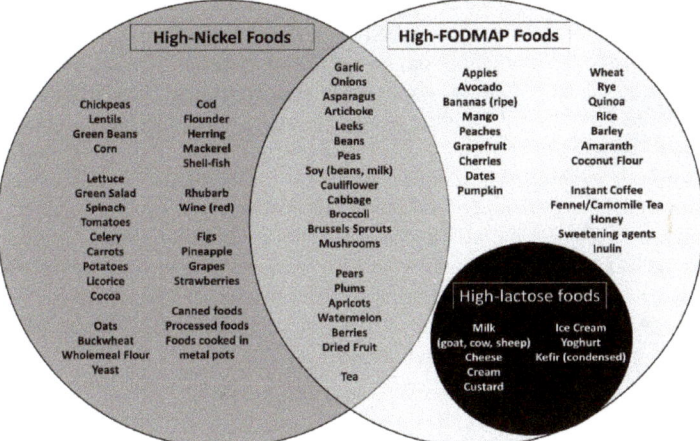

Figure 1. Foods with high nickel (Ni) content and their possible overlap with foods rich in fermentable oligo-, di-, and monosaccharides and polyols (FODMAPs). Here we report some of the main foods belonging to specific categories. To be noted is the overlap between Ni-rich foods and foods with high FODMAP content, as well as the overlap between foods high in FODMAPs and lactose content [10,15–19].

2. Materials and Methods

2.1. Patients

Study design: pilot study. We recruited 102 consecutive CD patients (74 female, 28 male; age range 18–65 years, mean age 42.3 ± 7.4) on a GFD since at least 12 months, with current serum EMA and anti-tTG antibodies negative results and histological remission (Marsh–Oberhuber type 0–I) who complained of relapsing or persisting gastrointestinal and/or extraintestinal symptoms. They referred to our Gastroenterology Unit from January 2017 to December 2019. Their CD diagnosis had been previously made according gluten-related signs and symptoms, serum EMA and anti-tTG antibodies positive results, and the histological finding of duodenal villous atrophy (Marsh–Oberhuber type IIIA, B, or C) [20–22].

Inclusion criteria: presence of at least three gastrointestinal symptoms with a score ≥5 on the modified GSRS questionnaire completed at study recruitment, in order to exclude patients with less significant clinical pictures. Exclusion criteria: IgE-mediated food allergy (diagnosed by skin prick test or laboratory tests (ImmunoCAP) for serum allergen-specific IgE antibodies); history of past or current cancer; inflammatory bowel disease; infectious diseases including *Helicobacter pylori* (HP); lactose intolerance (by means of the lactose breath test and genetic evaluation of lactase-gene polymorphism [23,24]).

The study was performed in compliance with the Declaration of Helsinki. Approval of the local ethics committee was obtained (study approval: report 8.2.0 06/2020 of the Board of the Department of Translational and Precision Medicine—Sapienza University of Rome). Written informed consent was obtained from all patients.

2.2. Symptom Questionnaire

The Gastrointestinal Symptom Rating Scale (GSRS) questionnaire modified according to "Salerno's experts' criteria" is a standardized tool used in the diagnostic protocol for non-celiac gluten sensitivity, and it has also been employed to objectively evaluate the clinical status in other IBS-like disorders such as Ni sensitivity [15]. It consists of a list of gastrointestinal and extraintestinal symptoms associated to a numeric scale (score ranging from 0 to 10), which represents the intensity perceived by the patients during a specific dietary regimen [25]. Gastrointestinal symptoms include abdominal pain, heartburn, acid regurgitation, bloating, nausea, borborygmus, swelling, belching, flatulence, decreased or increased evacuations, loose or hard stools, urgent need for defecation, oral/tongue ulcers. Extraintestinal symptoms include dermatitis, headache, foggy mind, fatigue, numbness of the limbs, joint/muscle pain, fainting [15].

According to our standard outpatient treatment protocol for the management of CD, the questionnaire had been previously administered at CD diagnosis (T0) and after at least 12 months of GFD, when serological and histological remission had been achieved (T1). After at least three further months on a GFD, a third questionnaire was administered to those CD patients who complained of a relapse of gastrointestinal and extraintestinal symptoms, despite confirmed negative serological and histological results to exclude refractory CD (T2, study recruitment). The last questionnaire was administered after 3 months of LNiD in addition to GFD (T3).

2.3. Nickel Oral Mucosa Patch Test

Once enrolled in the study (T2), all patients underwent an Ni omPT to detect the presence of Ni ACM. Ni omPT is a 5 mm filter paper disk saturated with a 5% solution of Ni sulfate in Vaseline (0.4 mg Ni-sulfate/8 mg Vaseline). It is applied on the upper lip mucosa and held in place by a transparent adhesive film (Tegaderm, 3M, St. Paul, MN - USA). For appropriate diagnostic purposes, a control test with only 8 mg Vaseline is also provided and applied. Local Ni-induced type IV hypersensitivity reactions (e.g., edema, hyperemia, aphthous/vesicular lesions) can be evident after just 2 h of exposure or even after 24–48 h as late reactions. Late general symptoms triggered by omPT (e.g., swelling, abdominal pain, diarrhea, headache, foggy mind, itching) should also be considered as positive test results [14,15].

2.4. Low-Nickel Diet

All enrolled patients followed a balanced GFD with the addition of an LNiD for 3 months after a visit with trained dieticians, who verified correct adherence to both diet regimens by means of a daily dietary diary and biweekly telephone interviews. Ni is an element abundantly present in many foods, with a certain concentration variability depending on the type of soil and plant species, irrigation water, fertilizers, and pesticides. Thus, since its total elimination from the diet is impossible, we recommended to avoid only foods with an estimated high content of Ni (Ni > 100 µg/kg) (Figure 1). The use of stainless-steel utensils and pots has also been discouraged, in order to reduce Ni contamination during cooking [15,19,26].

2.5. Statistical Analysis

Data obtained during the present study were both qualitative (omPT results) and quantitative (modified GSRS questionnaire). Qualitative data were expressed as frequencies (both absolute and relative). The symptoms' scores (GSRS scale: 0 = absent, 10 = maximum intensity) were summarized by median, and Wilcoxon's signed-rank test was used to compare each symptom at different times (T0, T1, T2, T3). Applying the Bonferroni correction, p-value <0.0083 (alpha = 0.05/6 comparisons) was considered statistically significant. Statistical analysis was performed using the Stata software, version 16.0 (Stata Cooperation, College Station, TX, USA).

Study arrangement and patient enrollment are summarized in Figure 2a,b.

Study management, Ni omPT, administration of the modified GSRS questionnaire, patient follow-up, and final data processing were performed at the Department of Translational and Precision Medicine.

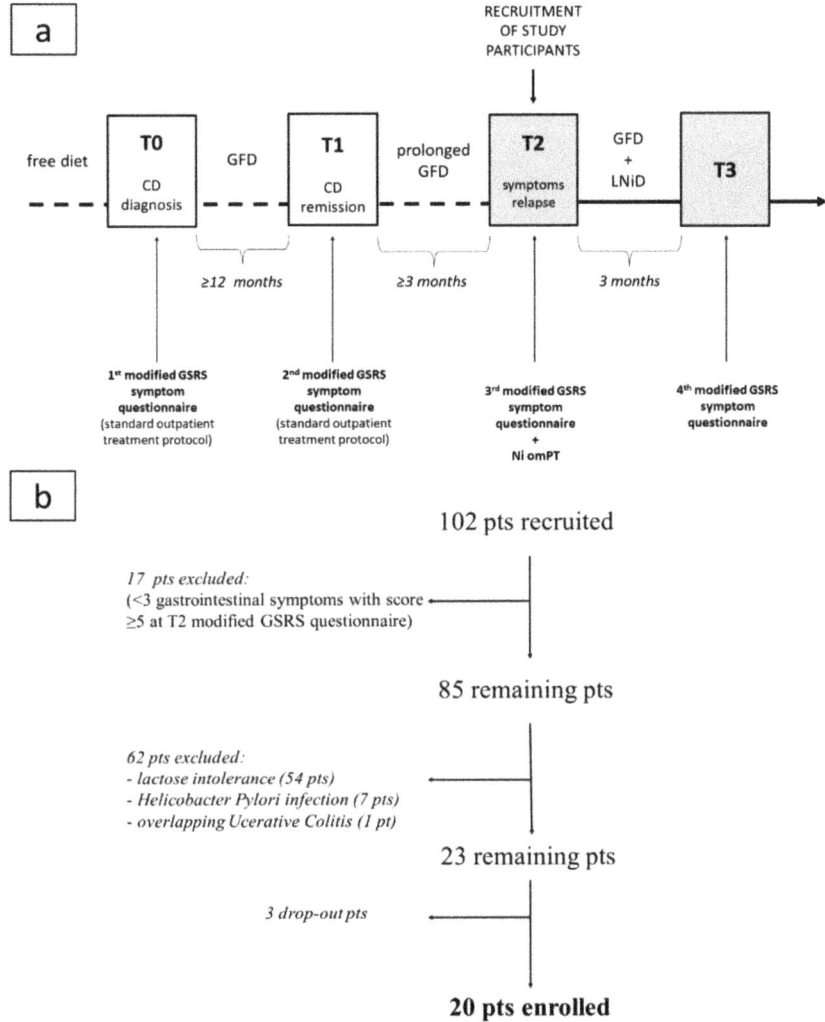

Figure 2. Flow charts of the study: (**a**) study arrangement; (**b**) patient enrollment. Legend: CD, celiac disease; GFD, gluten-free diet; GSRS, Gastrointestinal Symptom Rating Scale; LNiD, low-nickel diet; Ni omPT, nickel oral mucosa patch test; pts, patients.

3. Results

3.1. Patients

Of the 102 patients recruited, 17 patients were excluded since they did not meet the criterion of at least three gastrointestinal symptoms with a score ≥5 in the GSRS questionnaire completed at T2. Sixty-two out of the remaining 85 patients were also excluded: 54 were lactose intolerant, 7 were affected by HP infection, 1 was affected by overlapping active ulcerative colitis. Three out of the remaining 23 patients dropped out of the study, reporting that they no longer wanted to follow further food restrictions. Therefore, a total of 20 patients (all female, age range 23–65 years, mean age 39.1 ± 2.9, median age 40) completed the study (Figure 2b).

3.2. Nickel Oral Mucosa Patch Test

All 20 patients studied (100%) showed Ni omPT positive results and received an Ni ACM diagnosis. They all showed evident local mucosal alterations induced by Ni (erythema, edema, and/or vesicles) within 2 h after patch application (Figure 3a,b). What is more, all 20 patients showed at least one additional gastrointestinal or extraintestinal systemic symptom within 48 h after Ni omPT.

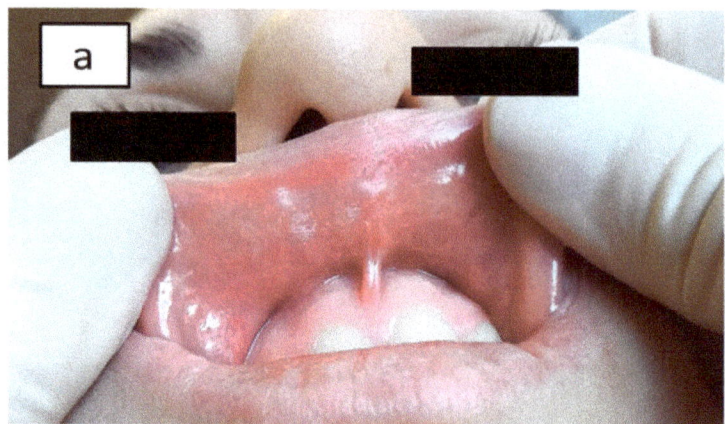

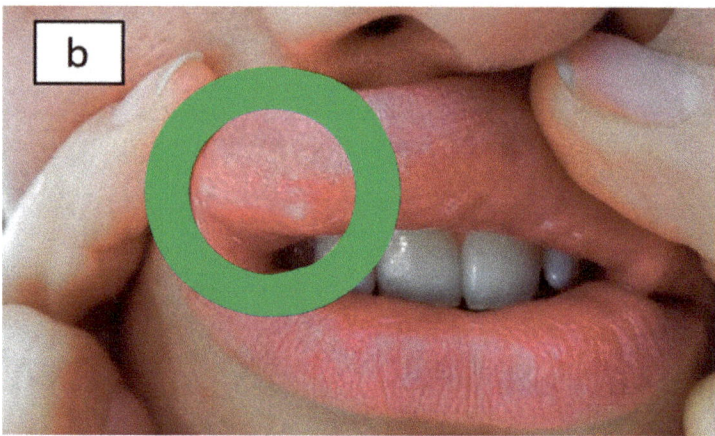

Figure 3. Nickel oral mucosa patch test (Ni omPT) results: Ni-sensitive patients before Ni omPT application (**a**) and after Ni omPT removal (2 h) (**b**).

3.3. Symptom Questionnaire

A correct GFD (T0 vs. T1) induced an improving trend in 19 out of the total 24 (79.2%) symptoms, and 14 out of 24 (58.3%) were statistically significant (p-value < 0.0083).

The prolonged GFD (T1 vs. T2) revealed a worsening trend in 20 out of the total 24 (83.3%) symptoms, and 10 out of 24 (41.7%) were statistically significant: abdominal pain, bloating, nausea, swelling, loose stools, dermatitis, fatigue, numbness of the limbs, and muscle and joint pain.

Once an Ni ACM diagnosis was obtained, an LNiD (T2 vs. T3) determined an improving trend in 20 out of the total 24 (83.4%) symptoms, and in 10 out of 24 (41.7%) symptoms the improvement was statistically significant. In detail, 12 out of 15 (80%) gastrointestinal symptoms improved, and 7 out of 15 (46.7%) showed a statistically significant improvement. In the same interval, 8 out of 9 (88.9%) extraintestinal symptoms showed an improvement, and 3 out of 9 (33.3%) significantly improved.

More details about gastrointestinal and extraintestinal symptoms during the different intervals analyzed are reported in Figures 4 and 5 and Table 1.

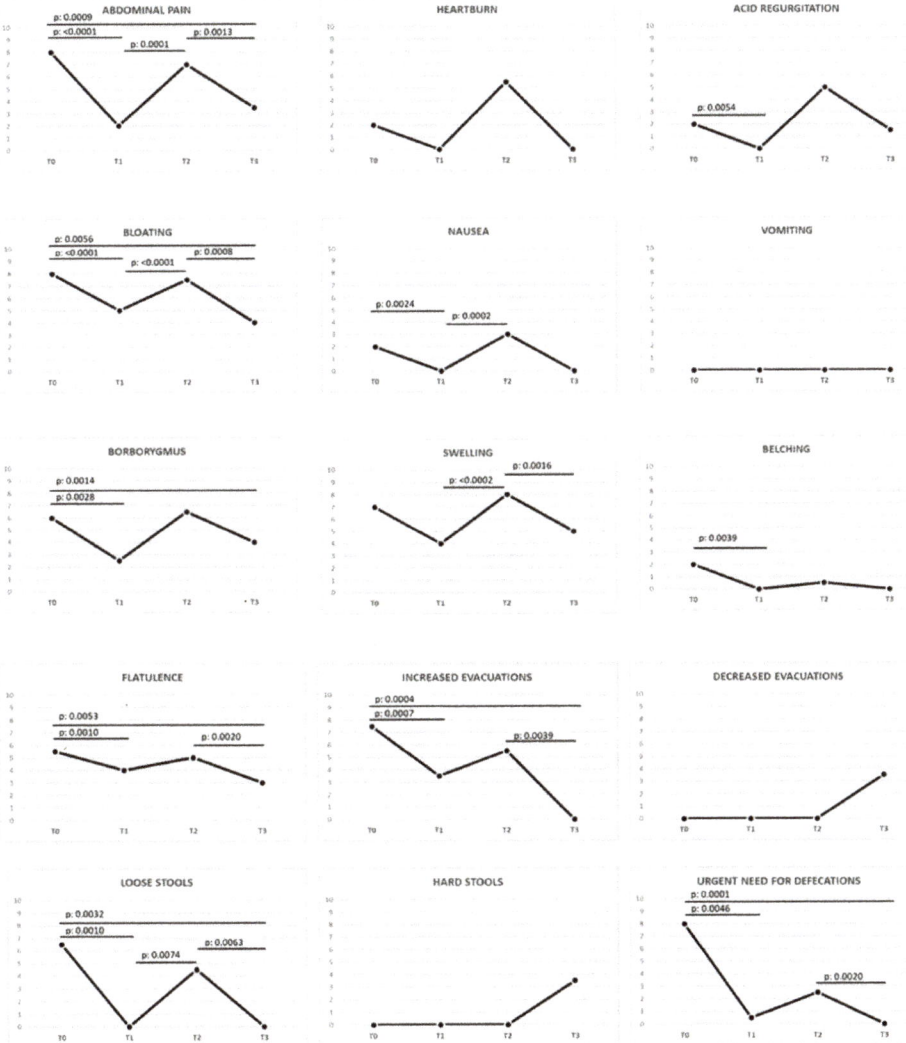

Figure 4. Variation of gastrointestinal symptoms in celiac patients during different stages of the study. The *p*-value was calculated using the Wilcoxon signed-rank test (statistically significant *p*-value < 0.0083

according to Bonferroni correction). Legend: GSRS, Gastrointestinal Symptom Rating Scale; T0, baseline, during gluten-containing diet; T1, after ≥12 months of proper gluten-free diet; T2, after ≥3 months of prolonged gluten-free and Ni-rich diet; T3, after 3 months of low-nickel and gluten-free diet.

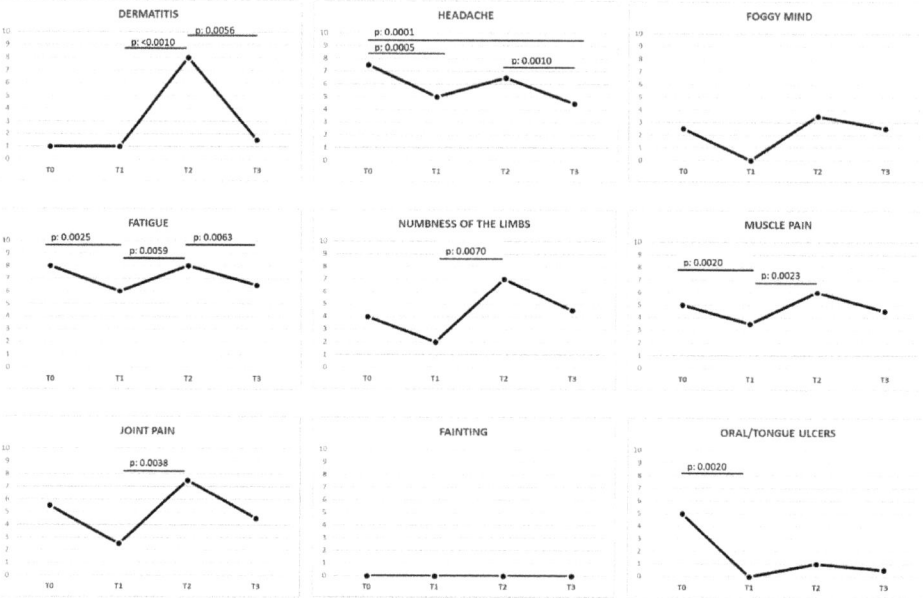

Figure 5. Variation of extraintestinal symptoms in celiac patients during different stages of the study. The *p*-value was calculated using the Wilcoxon signed-rank test (statistically significant *p*-value < 0.0083 according to Bonferroni correction). Legend: GSRS, Gastrointestinal Symptom Rating Scale; T0, baseline, during gluten-containing diet; T1, after ≥12 months of proper gluten-free diet; T2, after ≥3 months of prolonged gluten-free and nickel-rich diet; T3, after 3 months of low-nickel and gluten-free diet.

Table 1. Gastrointestinal and extra-intestinal symptoms during the different intervals analyzed. The table shows for each category of symptoms how many of them improved, worsened or remained stable in the different ranges of time considered. Data are reported in both absolute and percentage values. Legend: CD, celiac disease; GFD, gluten-free diet; LNiD, low nickel diet; n, number; Ni, Nickel; STAT. SIGN., statistically significant; tot, total; VS, versus.

	Comparison Description	Gastrointestinal Symptoms (tot n = 15)					Extra-Intestinal Symptoms (tot n = 9)					All Symptoms (tot n = 24)				
		Improvement		Worsening		Stability n (%)	Improvement		Worsening		Stability n (%)	Improvement		Worsening		Stability n (%)
		n (%)	Stat. Sign. n (%)	n (%)	Stat. Sign. n (%)		n (%)	Stat. Sign. n (%)	n (%)	Stat. Sign. n (%)		n (%)	Stat. Sign. n (%)	n (%)	Stat. Sign. n (%)	
T0 VS T1	CD remission achievement by GFD	12 (80%)	10 (66.7%)	0 (0%)	0 (0%)	3 (20%)	7 (77.8%)	4 (44.4%)	0 (0%)	0 (0%)	2 (22.2%)	19 (79.2%)	14 (58.3%)	0 (0%)	0 (0%)	5 (20.8%)
T1 VS T2	prolonged GFD (Ni load?)	0 (0%)	0 (0%)	12 (80%)	5 (33.3%)	3 (20%)	0 (0%)	0 (0%)	8 (88.9%)	5 (55.5%)	1 (11.1%)	0 (0%)	0 (0%)	20 (83.3%)	10 (41.7%)	4 (16.7%)
T2 VS T3	effects of LNiD during prolonged GFD	12 (80%)	7 (46.7%)	2 (13.3%)	0 (0%)	1 (6.7%)	8 (88.9%)	3 (33.3%)	0 (0%)	0 (0%)	1 (11.1%)	20 (83.4%)	10 (41.7%)	2 (8.3%)	0 (0%)	2 (8.3%)
T0 VS T2	active CD VS prolonged GFD (Ni load?)	7 (46.7%)	0 (0%)	5 (33.3%)	0 (0%)	3 (20%)	2 (22.2%)	0 (0%)	5 (55.6%)	0 (0%)	2 (22.2%)	9 (37.5%)	0 (0%)	10 (41.7%)	0 (0%)	5 (20.8%)
T0 VS T3	Active CD VS prolonged GFD + LNiD	12 (80%)	7 (46.7%)	2 (13.3%)	0 (0%)	1 (6.7%)	5 (55.6%)	1 (11.1%)	2 (22.2%)	0 (0%)	2 (22.2%)	17 (70.8%)	8 (33.3%)	4 (16.7%)	0 (0%)	3 (12.5%)
T1 VS T3	initial GFD VS prolonged GFD + LNiD	4 (26.7%)	0 (0%)	6 (40%)	0 (0%)	5 (33.3%)	1 (11.1%)	0 (0%)	7 (77.8%)	0 (0%)	1 (11.1%)	5 (20.8%)	0 (0%)	13 (54.2%)	0 (0%)	6 (25%)

4. Discussion

The persistence or recurrence of gastrointestinal and/or extraintestinal symptoms in CD patients during GFD is a very common condition and is a topic of great relevance. The causes of this problem are to be initially searched in an incorrect adherence to GFD and this is what can happen in those patients who still show persistently positive antibody titers and significant duodenal histological alterations, even despite quite a long period of GFD (>12 months). Furthermore, the possibility of refractory CD is always to be taken into consideration [4,6–8].

This issue becomes even more difficult to decipher and solve when CD patients reach serological and histological remission, but symptoms are still present or show a new peak despite a correct GFD. Furthermore, some of these patients may even report the appearance of new symptoms never complained about before. Other overlapping disorders, such as IBS or IBS-like disorders may be the causes of these symptoms and, in this regard, encouraging results have been obtained by ex adiuvantibus use of a low-FODMAP diet, although this approach revealed some limitations that will be discussed further [9,10].

On the other hand, many gluten-free foods consumed by CD patients are high in Ni content. Therefore, once a CD diagnosis has been obtained, the progressive Ni load induced by the GFD can trigger a relapse of symptoms in subjects predisposed to Ni allergy. Ni is present in many foods with different concentrations. It can be responsible for SNAS, which can have both gastrointestinal and extraintestinal manifestations. Specifically, Ni ACM is estimated to be one of the most common IBS-like disorders, and its diagnosis can rely on an Ni omPT, more sensitive and specific than the epicutaneous patch test [11]. What is more, excellent clinical results have already been obtained by Ni omPT and LNiD in the management of IBS-like and extraintestinal symptoms of women suffering from endometriosis who were still symptomatic despite different treatments [15,17].

Based on these considerations, we investigated the prevalence of Ni ACM in still symptomatic CD subjects after appropriate GFD and studied the effects of an LNiD on their gastrointestinal and extraintestinal symptoms.

Firstly, we selected symptomatic CD patients on a proper GFD who had no more serological and histological signs of disease activity. Then, we excluded those who did not meet the minimum clinical criterion by means of the GSRS questionnaire: in this way, we eliminated the less disabling and most confounding clinical pictures, even if this has led to a reduction in the number of patients studied. Other possible overlapping confounding pathologies have been excluded, such as lactose intolerance, HP infection and IBDs.

Our results showed an Ni ACM prevalence of 100% in the final 20 patients actually enrolled (Figure 3a,b): this percentage may appear extraordinarily high, but it is mandatory to consider not only the high prevalence of Ni ACM in the general population (estimated to be even greater than 30%) but also the strict exclusion criteria previously applied [11]. These 20 patients with Ni omPT positive results should be contextualized among the 85 CD patients who had a significant symptomatic picture: thus, Ni ACM should have a prevalence of at least 23.5% in our study. This percentage could have been higher considering not only the dropouts but also those patients affected by other pathologies who had been excluded in recruitment phase: in fact, Ni ACM can also easily overlap with other disorders, especially lactose intolerance, and in our study we excluded 54 lactose intolerant patients (about 63.5% of the 85 patients with a significant clinical picture) [11].

Afterward we focused on the effects of the different diet regimens on the symptoms.

First, we confirmed a general clinical improvement after CD diagnosis and a correct GFD (T0 vs. T1): once serological and histological remission were achieved, about 80% of the 24 total symptoms improved (almost 60% was also statistically significant).

On the other hand, a prolonged strict GFD (T1 vs. T2) resulted in a general clinical relapse involving more than 80% of all symptoms (the worsening was statistically significant in more than 40% of the symptoms). This negative change may be attributed to a GFD-related load of Ni in already sensitive or predisposed subjects.

This theory seemed to be confirmed after a balanced restriction of Ni-rich foods: in only three months, GFD plus LNiD (T2 vs. T3) induced an improvement of more than 80% of the symptoms and in the half of the cases the improvement was statistically significant, including the most complained about and disabling symptoms, such as abdominal pain, swelling, increased evacuations, and loose stools. Moreover, many of them got even better compared to the initial GFD alone (T1 vs. T3), although this difference was not statistically significant. As regards extraintestinal symptoms in the T2 vs. T3 range, dermatitis, headache, and fatigue statistically improved. Dermatitis deserves a special mention, as it showed a very peculiar trend: at the beginning (T0 and T1) it was almost totally absent, then it was significantly exacerbated reaching an acute peak at T2 and finally significantly reduced/resolved after GFD plus LNiD at T3. The curve of dermatitis' clinical course can further suggest the interference of an "alimentary trigger factor" during prolonged GFD, which is not related to gluten contamination, as demonstrated by the negative serological and histological results. The dietary profile of CD patients on a GFD and the impressive results of both Ni omPT and LNiD, would confirm that alimentary Ni overload is able to unmask/exacerbate not only gastrointestinal but also systemic symptoms, over a medium to long-term time period.

It should be emphasized that no symptoms significantly improved or worsened by comparing T0 (free diet) with T2 (Ni overload during GFD), suggesting a close clinical similarity between these two times: this is what often makes gastroenterologists think that the cause of the clinical relapse is a new gluten contamination.

The comparison between free diet and GFD + LNiD (T0 vs. T3) led to an improving trend of more than 70% of the symptoms: this is a very good percentage, although slightly lower than the almost 80% obtained from GFD alone, before Ni overload (T0 vs. T1). This may mean that, although LNiD is very effective in achieving a new clinical remission, Ni-sensitive patients cannot completely eliminate Ni, therefore, Ni-related symptoms, from their GFD.

The comparison between the well-being obtained by the initial GFD alone and the well-being obtained by the addition of the LNiD (T1 vs. T3) is also interesting: these two stages showed no statistically significant difference in symptoms' intensity perceived. This means that after the relapse peak in T2 (Ni load), a correct dietary intervention (LNiD) is able to completely restore well-being again.

The absence of a trial design was a limit of our study. Furthermore, it was carried out in a single center, the final sample size was quite small, and finally resulted in including only female patients. In addition, the very high prevalence of Ni omPT positive results (100%) may seem misleading.

Firstly, our results must be contextualized in the initial larger pool (102 total patients): the choice to exclude from the study those patients with less marked symptomatic pictures certainly led to the underdiagnosis of many other Ni-sensitive patients. In addition, it should be considered that Ni ACM can coexist with other disorders and can overlap with them from the symptomatic point of view [11]: in our study many HP-positive and lactose intolerant patients (almost 60% of the 102 patients initially recruited) were excluded for methodological correctness, and, thus, many other Ni-sensitive patients were probably lost among them.

The fact that the final 20 patients studied were only females is probably due to the greater prevalence of females in CD: in literature the female/male ratio is estimated to be about 3:1 and this proportion is approximately preserved in the 102 patients recruited at the beginning [27]. Furthermore, it has been described that Ni can act as a metalloestrogen and, thus, may have a greater influence in women with both extraintestinal and gastrointestinal clinical manifestations [15,28].

Given the strict differential diagnosis previously performed, this would explain such a high percentage (100%) of Ni omPT positive results. Moreover, the specific and successful treatment by LNiD seemed to confirm the appropriateness of our assumptions and supported the Ni omPT positive results: as above mentioned, more than 80% of symptoms improved after LNiD and about the half of them were statistically significant. In this regard, if we had not used the Bonferroni correction ($p < 0.05$ instead of $p < 0.0083$), the improvements of some other important symptoms (borborygmus, foggy mind, muscle pain, and joint pain) would have resulted statistically significant. We hope that future trials with larger populations will be able to confirm these preliminary observations.

Another weak point of our study, as well as possible obstacle for future trials, may be the impossibility to accurately measure Ni contained in foods and biological samples from patients studied. There is some variability of Ni content in foods and, to date, there are still no standard methods to measure it routinely: if these methods existed, we would have the possibility to prescribe highly personalized diets, more effectively monitor the intake of Ni-rich foods, and make even more appropriate comparisons. As recently demonstrated, we can successfully overcome this limit by prescribing patients a balanced LNiD on the base of an estimated average content of Ni in foods and under direct control of trained dieticians. A daily dietary diary and a detailed interview were also used to verify correct adherence to the GFD and LNiD.

It has already been described in literature that a low-FODMAP diet as an ex adiuvantibus treatment can benefit still symptomatic CD patients on a GFD. However, this dietary intervention has not so far been supported by specific diagnostic tests [9]. Moreover, it is known that many foods with estimated high content of FODMAPs may also cause other IBS-like disorders, such as lactose intolerance. It is therefore possible that during a low-FODMAP diet, other underlying and unrecognized diseases are treated. In this regard, we also observed a significant overlap between FODMAP-rich and Ni-rich foods (Figure 1), especially corn and other gluten-free foods consumed by CD subjects. It is therefore possible that the benefits of a low-FODMAP diet can depend on a concomitant involuntary LNiD in unrecognized Ni-sensitive patients. Given the high prevalence of Ni ACM and our results, this is more than only a hypothesis. On the other hand, our study can claim among its strengths an accurate preliminary differential diagnosis with other common IBS-like disorders and organic diseases. In addition, a targeted LNiD was prescribed after a reliable specific diagnostic test (Ni omPT), thus avoiding unnecessary dietary exclusions [15].

It may also be interesting to discuss the possible effects of close contact with patients during follow-up: frequent and extensive dietary interviews can have a placebo effect in clinical setting, capable even of inhibiting a symptom. On the other hand, they are essential methodological tools for an adequate quality assessment of the diet followed, as well as for the determination of the patient's clinical status. Close clinical contact also seemed to play a relevant role in supporting such "delicate" patients who had to follow two strict diet regimens: GFD and LNiD. This was confirmed not only by the encouraging clinical results obtained but also by the very low number of drop-outs. In addition, close clinical contact appeared even more necessary for such a study spread over a long period of time: the long time span of observation could have led to misestimation of the beneficial or harmful effects of dietary interventions. Finally, the inclusion of a significant number of symptoms in the GSRS standardized test for clinical evaluation has most probably helped to further reduce possible placebo/nocebo effects and misestimation of the results.

5. Conclusions

In conclusion, our findings show for the first time that Ni-rich foods and Ni ACM can frequently be the cause of relapsing gastrointestinal and extraintestinal symptoms in CD patients, even/especially during a correct GFD. Furthermore, our study not only confirms the usefulness of Ni omPT in making an Ni ACM diagnosis but also highlights that a balanced LNiD in addition to a correct GFD can offer a significant clinical improvement in this category of patients.

Further studies with larger populations should be carried out to confirm these important data, which may change the clinical management of CD patients.

Author Contributions: Conceptualization, R.B. and A.P.; data curation, R.B., N.D.A., and A.B.; formal analysis, R.B., N.D.A., A.B., N.G., and G.D.; investigation, R.B. and A.P.; methodology, R.B., A.B., and N.G.; project administration, R.B. and A.P.; software, A.B.; supervision, R.B., G.D., and A.P.; validation, R.B., G.D., and A.P.; visualization, R.B., N.G., and A.P.; writing—original draft, R.B.; writing—review and editing, R.B. and A.P. Guarantor of article: A.P. is the author who is acting as the submission's guarantor. All authors have read and agreed to the published version of the manuscript.

Funding: No institutional, private, or corporate financial support for the work was received. This research received no external funding.

Conflicts of Interest: The authors declare no conflict of interest.

References

1. Picarelli, A.; Borghini, R.; Isonne, C.; Di Tola, M. Reactivity to dietary gluten: New insights into differential diagnosis among gluten-related gastrointestinal disorders. *Pol. Arch. Med. Wewn.* **2013**, *123*, 708–712. [CrossRef]
2. Murray, J.A.; Frey, M.R.; Oliva-Hemker, M. Celiac Disease. *Gastroenterology* **2018**, *154*, 2005–2008. [CrossRef] [PubMed]
3. Lebwohl, B.; Sanders, D.S.; Green, P.H.R. Coeliac disease. *Lancet* **2018**, *391*, 70–81. [CrossRef]
4. Elli, L.; Ferretti, F.; Orlando, S.; Vecchi, M.; Monguzzi, E.; Roncoroni, L.; Schuppan, D. Management of celiac disease in daily clinical practice. *Eur. J. Intern. Med.* **2019**, *61*, 15–24. [CrossRef] [PubMed]
5. Picarelli, A.; Borghini, R.; Marino, M.; Casale, R.; Di Tola, M.; Lubrano, C.; Piermattei, A.; Gualdi, G.; Bella, A.; Donato, G.; et al. Visceral and subcutaneous adipose tissue as markers of local and systemic inflammation: A comparison between celiac and obese patients using MRI. *Tech. Coloproctol.* **2020**, *24*, 553–562. [CrossRef]
6. Laurikka, P.; Salmi, T.; Collin, P.; Huhtala, H.; Mäki, M.; Kaukinen, K.; Kurppa, K. Gastrointestinal Symptoms in Celiac Disease Patients on a Long-Term Gluten-Free Diet. *Nutrients* **2016**, *8*, 429. [CrossRef]
7. Husby, S.; Murray, J.A.; Katzka, D.A. AGA Clinical Practice Update on Diagnosis and Monitoring of Celiac Disease-Changing Utility of Serology and Histologic Measures: Expert Review. *Gastroenterology* **2019**, *156*, 885–889. [CrossRef]
8. Penny, H.A.; Baggus, E.M.R.; Rej, A.; Snowden, J.A.; Sanders, D.S. Non-Responsive Coeliac Disease: A Comprehensive Review from the NHS England National Centre for Refractory Coeliac Disease. *Nutrients* **2020**, *12*, 216. [CrossRef]
9. Roncoroni, L.; Bascuñán, K.A.; Doneda, L.; Scricciolo, A.; Lombardo, V.; Branchi, F.; Ferretti, F.; Dell'Osso, B.; Montanari, V.; Bardella, M.T.; et al. A Low FODMAP Gluten-Free Diet Improves Functional Gastrointestinal Disorders and Overall Mental Health of Celiac Disease Patients: A Randomized Controlled Trial. *Nutrients* **2018**, *10*, 1023. [CrossRef]
10. Varney, J.; Barrett, J.; Scarlata, K.; Catsos, P.; Gibson, P.R.; Muir, J.G. FODMAPs: Food composition, defining cutoff values and international application. *J. Gastroenterol. Hepatol.* **2017**, *32* (Suppl. 1), 53–61. [CrossRef]
11. Borghini, R.; Donato, G.; Alvaro, D.; Picarelli, A. New insights in IBS-like disorders: Pandora's box has been opened; a review. *Gastroenterol. Hepatol. Bed. Bench.* **2017**, *10*, 79–89. [PubMed]
12. Di Tola, M.; Marino, M.; Amodeo, R.; Tabacco, F.; Casale, R.; Portaro, L.; Borghini, R.; Cristaudo, A.; Manna, F.; Rossi, A.; et al. Immunological characterization of the allergic contact mucositis related to the ingestion of nickel-rich foods. *Immunobiology* **2014**, *219*, 522–530. [CrossRef] [PubMed]
13. Pazzini, C.A.; Pereira, L.J.; Marques, L.S.; Generoso, R.; de Oliveira, G., Jr. Allergy to nickel in orthodontic patients: Clinical and histopathologic evaluation. *Gen Dent.* **2010**, *58*, 58–61. [PubMed]
14. Borghini, R.; Puzzono, M.; Rosato, E.; Di Tola, M.; Marino, M.; Greco, F.; Picarelli, A. Nickel-Related Intestinal Mucositis in IBS-Like Patients: Laser Doppler Perfusion Imaging and Oral Mucosa Patch Test in Use. *Biol. Trace. Elem. Res.* **2016**, *173*, 55–61. [CrossRef] [PubMed]
15. Borghini, R.; Porpora, M.G.; Casale, R.; Marino, M.; Palmieri, E.; Greco, N.; Donato, G.; Picarelli, A. Irritable Bowel Syndrome-Like Disorders in Endometriosis: Prevalence of Nickel Sensitivity and Effects of a Low-Nickel Diet. An Open-Label Pilot Study. *Nutrients* **2020**, *12*, 341. [CrossRef]
16. Rizzi, A.; Nucera, E.; Laterza, L.; Gaetani, E.; Valenza, V.; Corbo, G.M.; Inchingolo, R.; Buonomo, A.; Schiavino, D.; Gasbarrini, A. Irritable Bowel Syndrome and Nickel Allergy: What Is the Role of the Low Nickel Diet? *J. Neurogastroenterol. Motil.* **2017**, *23*, 101–108. [CrossRef]
17. Lombardi, F.; Fiasca, F.; Minelli, M.; Maio, D.; Mattei, A.; Vergallo, I.; Cifone, M.G.; Cinque, B.; Minelli, M. The Effects of Low-Nickel Diet Combined with Oral Administration of Selected Probiotics on Patients with Systemic Nickel Allergy Syndrome (SNAS) and Gut Dysbiosis. *Nutrients* **2020**, *12*, 1040. [CrossRef]
18. Babaahmadifooladi, M.; Jacxsens, L.; Van de Wiele, T.; Laing, G.D. Gap analysis of nickel bioaccessibility and bioavailability in different food matrices and its impact on the nickel exposure assessment. *Food Res. Int.* **2020**, *129*, 108866. [CrossRef]

19. Braga, M.; Quecchia, C.; Perotta, C.; Timpini, A.; Maccarinelli, K.; Di Tommaso, L.; Di Gioacchino, M. Systemic nickel allergy syndrome: Nosologic framework and usefulness of diet regimen for diagnosis. *Int. J. Immunopathol. Pharmacol.* **2013**, *26*, 707–716. [CrossRef]
20. Al-Toma, A.; Volta, U.; Auricchio, R.; Castillejo, G.; Sanders, D.S.; Cellier, C.; Mulder, C.J.; Lundin, K.E.A. European Society for the Study of Coeliac Disease (ESsCD) guideline for coeliac disease and other gluten-related disorders. *United Eur. Gastroenterol. J.* **2019**, *7*, 583–613. [CrossRef]
21. Di Tola, M.; Marino, M.; Goetze, S.; Casale, R.; Di Nardi, S.; Borghini, R.; Donato, G.; Tiberti, A.; Picarelli, A. Identification of a serum transglutaminase threshold value for the noninvasive diagnosis of symptomatic adult celiac disease patients: A retrospective study. *J. Gastroenterol.* **2016**, *51*, 1031–1039. [CrossRef] [PubMed]
22. Khalesi, M.; Jafari, S.A.; Kiani, M.; Picarelli, A.; Borghini, R.; Sadeghi, R.; Eghtedar, A.; Ayatollahi, H.; Kianifar, H.R. In Vitro Gluten Challenge Test for Celiac Disease Diagnosis. *J. Pediatr. Gastroenterol. Nutr.* **2016**, *62*, 276–283. [CrossRef] [PubMed]
23. Usai-Satta, P.; Scarpa, M.; Oppia, F.; Cabras, F. Lactose malabsorption and intolerance: What should be the best clinical management? *World J. Gastrointest. Pharmacol. Ther.* **2012**, *3*, 29–33. [CrossRef] [PubMed]
24. Coluccia, E.; Iardino, P.; Pappalardo, D.; Brigida, A.L.; Formicola, V.; De Felice, B.; Guerra, C.; Pucciarelli, A.; Amato, M.R.; Riegler, G.; et al. Congruency of Genetic Predisposition to Lactase Persistence and Lactose Breath Test. *Nutrients* **2019**, *11*, 1383. [CrossRef]
25. Catassi, C.; Elli, L.; Bonaz, B.; Bouma, G.; Carroccio, A.; Castillejo, G.; Cellier, C.; Cristofori, F.; de Magistris, L.; Dolinsek, J.; et al. Diagnosis of Non-Celiac Gluten Sensitivity (NCGS): The Salerno Experts' Criteria. *Nutrients* **2015**, *7*, 4966–4977. [CrossRef] [PubMed]
26. Di Gioacchino, M.; Ricciardi, L.; De Pità, O.; Minelli, M.; Patella, V.; Voltolini, S.; Di Rienzo, V.; Braga, M.; Ballone, E.; Mangifesta, R.; et al. Nickel oral hyposensitization in patients with systemic nickel allergy syndrome. *Ann. Med.* **2014**, *46*, 31–37. [CrossRef] [PubMed]
27. Thomas, H.J.; Ahmad, T.; Rajaguru, C.; Barnardo, M.; Warren, B.F.; Jewell, D.P. Contribution of histological, serological, and genetic factors to the clinical heterogeneity of adult-onset coeliac disease. *Scand. J. Gastroenterol.* **2009**, *44*, 1076–1083. [CrossRef]
28. Aquino, N.B.; Sevigny, M.B.; Sabangan, J.; Louie, M.C. The role of cadmium and nickel in estrogen receptor signaling and breast cancer: Metalloestrogens or not? *J. Environ. Sci. Health C Environ. Carcinog. Ecotoxicol. Rev.* **2012**, *30*, 189–224. [CrossRef]

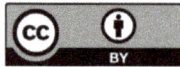

© 2020 by the authors. Licensee MDPI, Basel, Switzerland. This article is an open access article distributed under the terms and conditions of the Creative Commons Attribution (CC BY) license (http://creativecommons.org/licenses/by/4.0/).

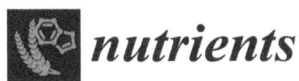

Article

Efficacy of a High-Iron Dietary Intervention in Women with Celiac Disease and Iron Deficiency without Anemia: A Clinical Trial

Alice Scricciolo [1,*], Luca Elli [1,2], Luisa Doneda [3], Karla A Bascunan [4], Federica Branchi [1,2], Francesca Ferretti [1,2], Maurizio Vecchi [1,2] and Leda Roncoroni [1,3]

[1] Center for Prevention and Diagnosis of Coeliac Disease-Gastroenterology and Endoscopy Unit, Fondazione IRCCS Ca' Granda Ospedale Maggiore Policlinico, Via F. Sforza 35, 20122 Milan, Italy; lucelli@yahoo.com (L.E.); federica.branchi@gmail.com (F.B.); francesca.ferretti01@gmail.com (F.F.); maurizio.vecchi@unimi.it (M.V.); leda.roncoroni@unimi.it (L.R.)
[2] Department of Pathophisiology and Transplantation, University of Milan, 20122 Milan, Italy
[3] Department of Biomedical, Surgical and Dental Sciences, University of Milan, 20122 Milan, Italy; luisa.doneda@unimi.it
[4] Department of Nutrition, School of Medicine, University of Chile, 8380453 Santiago, Chile; karlabascunan@gmail.com
* Correspondence: alice.scricciolo@policlinico.mi.it

Received: 17 June 2020; Accepted: 14 July 2020; Published: 17 July 2020

Abstract: Background and Aim. Iron deficiency without anemia (IDWA) is a common finding in celiac disease (CD) and can also persist in case of good compliance and clinical response to a strict gluten-free diet (GFD). This scenario usually presents in CD women of child-bearing age in whom the imbalance between menstrual iron loss and inadequate iron intake from their diet plays the major role. A recommended approach to this condition is yet to be established. This study aimed to compare, in this subset of patients, the efficacy of a dietary approach consisting of an iron-rich diet against the traditional pharmacological oral-replacement therapy. Material and Methods. Between February and December 2016, consecutive CD female patients of child-bearing age as referred to our outpatient center with evidence of IDWA (ferritin <15 ng/mL or 15–20 ng/L with transferrin saturation <15%) were enrolled. After the completion of a 7-day weighed food intake recording to assess the usual iron dietary intake, the patients were randomized in two arms to receive a 12-week iron-rich diet (iron intake >20 mg/die) versus oral iron supplementation with ferrous sulfate (FS) (105 mg/day). Blood tests and dietary assessments were repeated at the end of treatment. The degree of compliance and tolerability to the treatments were assessed every month by means of specific questionnaires and symptoms evaluation. Results. A total of 22 women were enrolled and divided in the diet group ($n = 10$, age 37 ± 8 years) and in the FS group ($n = 12$, age 38 ± 10 years). The food intake records demonstrated an inadequate daily intake of iron in all the enrolled subjects. At the end of the treatments, ferritin levels were higher in the FS group (8.5 (5) versus 34 (30.8), $p = 0.002$). Compliance and tolerability were similar in both treatment groups (89% versus 87%, $p = $ ns). Conclusions. These findings did not support any equivalent efficacy of an iron-rich diet compared to a FS supplementation in non-anemic iron-deficient women affected by CD. However, the diet appeared a well-tolerated approach, and adequate dietary instructions could effectively increase the daily iron consumption, suggesting a role in the long-term management of IDWA, especially in patients who do not tolerate pharmacological supplementation.

Keywords: Celiac disease; iron deficiency without anemia; dietary iron; iron supplementation; gluten-free diet; women

1. Introduction

Celiac disease (CD) is an autoimmune disorder that occurs in genetically predisposed individuals who develop an immune reaction to gluten [1]. In the Western countries, the prevalence has reached 1:100, with a male/female ratio 1/3 [2,3]. The CD hallmark consists in a damage of the gastrointestinal tract characterized by inflammation of the lamina propria, villous atrophy, crypt hyperplasia, and T-cell infiltration [4]. The clinical manifestations of CD are heterogeneous. The classic ones involve gastrointestinal-related symptoms due to malabsorption, mainly diarrhea and weight loss, but up to 30% of patients are asymptomatic. Furthermore, CD patients may present extra-intestinal symptoms, including mineral and vitamin deficiency. The most common mineral deficiencies are: iron-deficiency anemia (IDA) and iron-deficiency without anemia (IDWA) [5–8].

IDA is the most frequently sign observed in patients affected by CD, and different studies have shown that IDA can be the only symptom of CD [8–10]. Although not completely clear, iron deficiency (ID) in CD can be caused by malabsorption due to small bowel (SB) atrophy, which is a systemic inflammatory state and possible genetic variants. While most of the studies focalized on IDA, little is known about IDWA. Gluten-free diet (GFD) is able to restore intestinal trophism in the majority of patients, re-establishing the correct absorption of dietary iron [11] and reducing the cytokine levels. However, in spite of the intestinal mucosa normalization and clinical responsiveness, in a group of CD patients, IDWA may persist. Frequently, these patients are women of child-bearing age with menstrual blood losses and a subsequently progressive depletion of iron reserves. In the case of IDA, the current recommendations are to take pharmacological iron supplementation, in order to prevent the depletion of the iron deposits. It has been observed that the normalization of hemoglobin levels requires up to two years of therapy [12]. Experts do not recommend any specific treatment to IDWA patients, and there are no guidelines on this issue; consequently, it is unclear if this group of patients should be pharmacologically treated as in the case of IDA. Providing high doses of iron could not be a correct strategy in this group; in fact, iron overload may induce such negative effects as the formation of free radicals and protein and DNA damages [13,14]. Conversely, to increase the iron dietary intake changes in gluten-free diet (GFD) can restore iron deposits. From this point of view, the daily amount of iron recommended by the World Health Organization (WHO) varies according to the age and sex of individuals, being around 20 mg per day for women [15].

The aim of our clinical trial was to evaluate the efficacy of a high-iron gluten-free diet (GFD-HI) as compared to an oral iron therapy (ferrous sulfate) in a group of women affected by CD with IDWA.

2. Patients and Design

Our study patients were recruited at the "Center for Prevention and Diagnosis of Celiac Disease", Fondazione IRCCS Ca' Granda Ospedale Maggiore Policlinico in Milan between 1 February and 31 December 2016. CD diagnosis was based in accordance with the national and international guidelines [8]. Celiac adult women of pre-menopausal age, following a correct GFD for at least 1 year, presenting with IDWA (defined as ferritin levels <15 ng/L or ferritin 15–20 ng/L and transferrin saturation <15%), were enrolled.

The study was a prospective two-arm single-center randomized open-label trial. At enrolment (t0), the patients' demographic and clinical data were recorded; furthermore, a 7-day food diary was kept in order to verify the iron dietary intake. Blood tests including Hb, ferritin, iron, transferrin, anti tissue transglutaminase antibody were performed, and gastrointestinal symptoms were evaluated by means of 10-cm-long visual analogic scales (VAS). After these evaluations, the subjects were divided in two treatment arms for 12 weeks: (1) patients receiving a GFD with high-iron content, >20 mg per day; (2) patients receiving ferrous sulfate (FS) (105 mg/day, 1 oral tablet). The subjects were assigned to either treatment group on the basis of a randomization list generated by computer. All the patients were evaluated by a gastroenterologist and a qualified nutritionist: both experts in CD management. At the end of the treatment (t3), the patient's blood tests, gastrointestinal symptoms (VAS), and 7-day food diary were acquired. After 4 and 8 weeks from the beginning of their treatment, the patients were contacted by telephone in order to ascertain their adherence to the treatments and symptoms. The study flowchart has been reported in Figure 1.

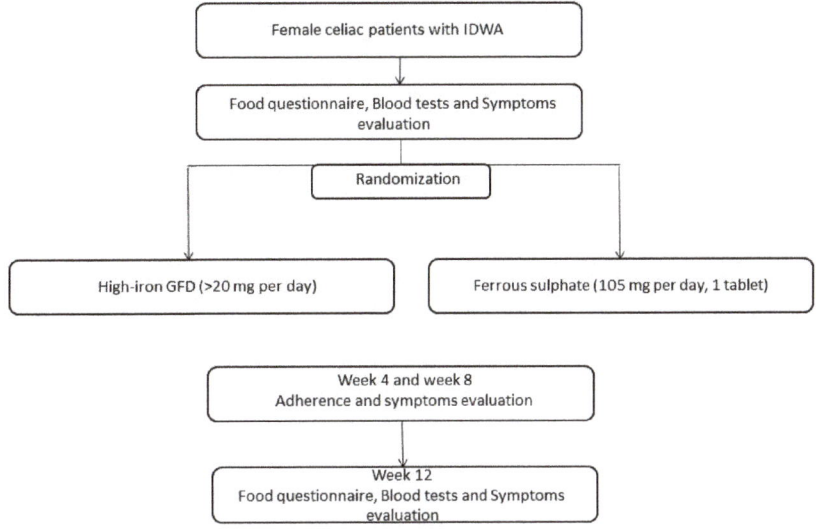

Figure 1. Flowchart of the study (*n* = 22).

The study was registered on http://clinicaltrials.gov/ (ref. no. NCT02949765). The University of Milan's Institutional Review Board checked and approved the study protocol according to the Helsinki Declaration, the Project Identification Code of the Local Ethics Committee's Approval of our study being 744_2015bis. The protocol was approved by the Ethics Committee of Milan/Area B on 14 January 2016). All the patients gave and signed their informed consent prior to participation in this study.

High-Iron Gluten-Free Diet

The subjects underwent an interview with a qualified nutritionist about the content and bio-availability of iron in the different foods. Foods were divided into three categories depending on their iron content (high, medium, and low), as identified by a previous study [16]. The quantity of iron contained in each food was determined via the Italian food composition tables [17]. The types of gluten-free (GF) foods in each category are shown in Supplementary Table S1. A nutritionally balanced GFD was designed with a combination of animal and vegetable food sources. The patients were advised to eat meals with a high intake of vitamin C to increase the absorption of iron, to limit fiber and avoid coffee, tea, or milk near mealtimes, in order to preserve a regular iron absorption [18–20]. To choose a diet with high-iron content, the patients were recommended to select one of the following four daily food combinations, with a specific number of portions per category: 1 high + 2 medium + 2 low, 1 high + 1 medium + 4 low, 4 medium + 2 low, 3 medium + 4 low. Each combination of foods ensured an intake of at least 20 mg/day iron. To verify the effective compliance with the assigned diet, the patients received questionnaires to be completed 15 times over the study period, about the daily food combination and about the advices to increase the absorption of iron.

3. Statistical Analysis

The data were described as median (interquartile range). The data distribution was assessed by graphical inspection and the Shapiro–Wilk test. Wilcoxon matched-pairs signed-ranks test used to compare iron status and gastrointestinal symptoms were reported by the patients within the groups before and after intervention. A Wilcoxon rank-sum test was used to compare gastrointestinal symptoms at the end of the intervention between groups. The VAS score for gastrointestinal symptoms before and after the intervention were analyzed by Analysis of Variance (ANOVA, including factors 'group' and 'time') for repeated measures ('time'). A 5% significance level was used, and the software packages STATA® v. 13.1 (StataCorp LLC, College Station, TX, USA) and GraphPad Prism v. 6 (GraphPad Software, La Jolla, CA, USA) were used for analysis and graphs processing.

4. Results

Twenty-two CD women with IDWA were enrolled and allocated to the GFD-HI group ($n = 10$, age 37 ± 8, mean age at diagnosis 27.1 ± 11.5) and to the FS group ($n = 12$, age 38 ± 10, mean age at diagnosis 29.3 ± 16). At enrolment, most of the patients (77.3%) presented with an insufficient iron dietary intake (7.37 ± 2.27 mg/day).

Hematological data at enrolment and at the end of treatment are reported in Table 1. It is appreciated that the pharmacological treatment significantly improved all blood parameters regarding the iron status. However, in the case of the GFD-HI group, the values at the end of intervention did not show an increase in iron indicators, showing only a tendency to improve ferritin levels in the women following a GFD-HI.

Table 1. Blood tests of the enrolled patients.

	GFD-HI Group ($n = 10$)			FS Group ($n = 12$)		
	t0	t3	p	t0	t3	p
Ferritin (ng/mL)	9 (4)	9 (5.2)	0.26	8.5 (5)	34 (30.8)	0.002
Hemoglobin (g/dL)	12.9 (0.4)	12.9 (1.2)	0.72	12.9 (0.6)	13.8 (1.0)	0.03
Iron (mcg/dL)	59 (53)	61 (58)	0.46	51 (37)	98 (27.5)	0.03
Transferrin (mg/dL)	314 (51)	300 (72)	0.06	304 (75.5)	256.5 (32.5)	0.002
Transferrin saturation (%)	14 (6)	10 (13)	0.14	12 (9.5)	24.5 (11)	0.007

Data described as median (interquartile range). Wilcoxon matched-pairs signed-ranks test was used to compare iron status within the groups before and after intervention. t0: enrolment, t3: 12 weeks, GFD-HI group: gluten-free diet with high-iron content group, FS group: ferrous sulfate group.

Regarding gastrointestinal symptoms, there were no significant differences when comparing the start and end of treatment in both groups (Table 2). However, it should be noted that for the FS group, there was a statistical tendency to high frequency of diarrhea around the start of the intervention.

Table 2. Gastrointestinal symptoms reported by the patients during the treatments.

	GFD-HI Group ($n = 10$)			FS Group ($n = 12$)			P †GFD-HI vs. FS at t3
	t0	t3	P *	t0	t3	P *	
Abdominal pain	0 (3)	0 (1)	0.85	0 (1.5)	0.5 (2)	0.35	0.581
Epigastric burning	0 (-)	0 (-)	-	0.5 (4)	0 (2.5)	0.58	0.056
Abdominal bloating	4 (5)	1 (4)	0.22	2.5 (5.5)	0.5 (4)	0.10	0.964
Diarrhea	0 (0)	0 (0)	0.31	0 (0)	0 (2)	0.04	0.300
Constipation	0 (0)	1 (5)	0.28	0 (4)	0 (5)	1.0	0.547

* Data described as median (interquartile range). Wilcoxon matched-pairs signed-ranks test used to compare gastrointestinal symptoms reported by the patients within the groups before and after intervention. † Wilcoxon rank sum test was used to compared gastrointestinal symptoms at the end of the intervention between group. t0: enrolment, t3: 12 weeks, GFD-HI group: gluten-free diet with high-iron content group, FS group: ferrous sulfate group.

Compliance and tolerability were similar in both treatments, with no patients suspending or interrupting the study (data not shown). The VAS scores regarding the symptoms reported by the patients during the trial are shown in Table 2 and Supplementary Figure S1.

5. Discussion

The present study is the first one evaluating the effectiveness of a GFD-HI in patients affected by CD and IDWA. The results of the study have shown that prescribing a diet with high iron content, although not sufficient to normalize the ferritin values in a group of CD women of child-bearing age, is still able to stabilize the levels of Hb, ferritin, and transferrin saturation, while previous studies on other groups of patients reported positive results, suggesting a non-inferiority of high-iron dieting compared to FS administration, especially on long-term observation [16]. On the other side, FS is a validated treatment with proven efficacy on iron deficiency, and the daily food intake is about 1/10th of the quantity present in the drug. Furthermore, in our study, the FS supplementation has been well tolerated, and the analysis of symptoms demonstrated only a slight, non-significant decrease of VAS in the GFD-HI group as compared to the FS group.

While the international guidelines mainly deal with IDA, the diagnostic and therapeutic approach it is not clear in case of IDWA [21]. Treating this condition might play a preventive role, especially in women of child-bearing age, as such women are exposed to the risk of developing IDA, because of the menstrual blood loss. However, oral iron supplementation can cause side effects and lead to the development of symptoms. In this study, the prescription of a GFD-HI involved a group of young women affected by CD. Generally, CD patients are more exposed to nutrients deficiency even after a correct GFD. Their iron deficiency in CD can be attributed to malabsorption, resulting from the persistence of villous atrophy, dietary mistakes, or the presence of genetic polymorphisms that limit iron absorption [22]. In addition, the use of GF industrially manufactured products has been reported to limit the intake of micronutrients as compared to the diet of the general population [23,24]. Iron is necessary for the proper functioning of different cellular mechanisms, including enzymatic processes, DNA synthesis, and mitochondrial energy production. The body of an adult contains 3–5 g iron, 20–25 mg are needed on a daily basis for the production of red blood cells and for cellular metabolism [25]. About 1–2 mg iron is lost daily because of epithelial desquamation, sweating, urinary secretion, and menstrual flow in women. Losses are usually balanced by the intestinal absorption of iron taken through diet and metabolic recycling [26]. The daily intake in milligrams of iron recommended by the World Health Organization (WHO) varies according to the age and sex of individuals, being ca. 20 mg per day for women [15]. A diet with high iron favors foods of animal source such as meat, offal, fish, seafood [27]. It was also advised to take such vegetable-based foods as legumes (beans, chickpeas, lentils), dried fruits (pistachios, cashew nuts, peanuts, dried apricots) and such other foods as rocket, dark chocolate, buckwheat, and olives, although their iron bio-availability is less than foods of animal source [28]. Furthermore, it was recommended to take fruit and vegetables rich in vitamin C such as kiwi, strawberries, citrus fruit, currants, papaya, red and yellow peppers, broccoli, cauliflower, and parsley at mealtimes, thanks to the potential of the ascorbic acid therein contained to favor the absorption of iron [18]. On the contrary, it was not recommended to take coffee, tea, or milk near mealtime, as their content in phenolic compounds (e.g., phytates, oxalates) and calcium may reduce iron absorption [19,29]. It was also advised to limit fiber intake, as fiber interferes with the regular absorption of iron [20]. On analyzing the 7-day food diaries of the enrolled patients, it showed that most patients did not present a sufficient iron intake through their diets.

In case of IDWA, the appropriate intervention is to ensure an adequate daily intake of iron that is sufficient to compensate its consumption. The choice of a therapeutic diet as an alternative to oral iron supplementation appears to be a potentially adequate option for patients with CD. In fact, they often have gastrointestinal symptoms [30], so the prescription of drugs with potential gastrointestinal effects (such as FS, currently considered as the standard therapy for ID and IDA) may be poorly tolerated or even contraindicated.

To achieve significant improvements with the diet in serum ferritin requires time (over nine months), so future studies need longer investigate times. In conclusion, the results of our pilot randomized trial on the efficacy of the GFD-HI in women of child-bearing age with CD do not currently allow for comparable efficacy between a high-iron diet over 12 weeks and the reference standard, i.e., the FS therapy. However, the diet was well tolerated and accepted by celiac patients, maintaining stable iron parameters and blocking any decreasing tendency. For this group of IDWA patients, it would be helpful to test a "run-in period" of 3 weeks of ferrous sulfate supplementation to stabilize their iron profiles and to recommend a high-iron diet that can be followed in the long-term, maintaining the iron blood values as stable (see Figure 2). Further data is expected from the long-term observation of the groups of patients enrolled, in order to highlight an effect on dietary habits, on the effective daily food intake of iron and on the effect of these changes on the iron profile. The support of expert nutritionists in the management of patients with CD appears indispensable not only to ensure an optimal approach to GFD, but also to identify early signs of malnutrition or malabsorption and to provide specific support in the adoption of correct eating habits toward the prevention of micronutrient deficiency, to which celiac subjects are particularly predisposed.

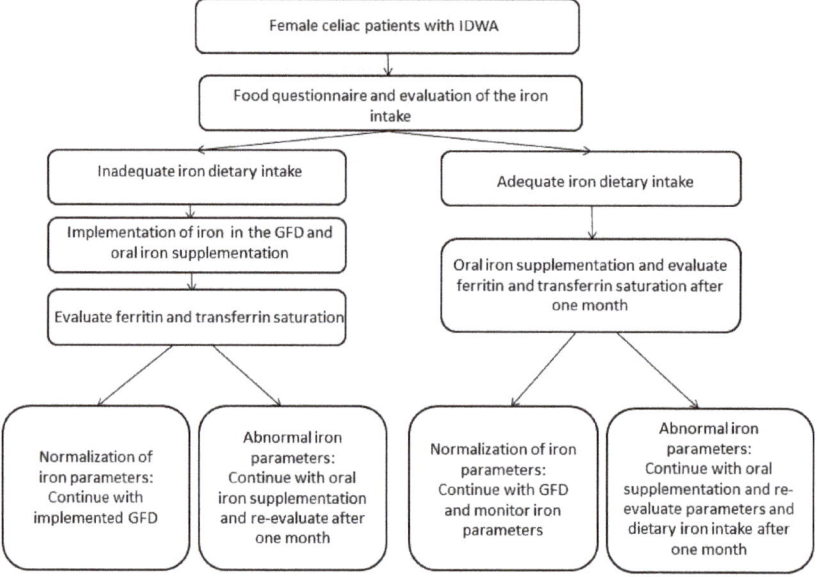

Figure 2. Roadmap in case of iron deficiency without anemia (IDWA) and celiac disease (CD).

Supplementary Materials: The following are available online at http://www.mdpi.com/2072-6643/12/7/2122/s1, Figure S1: Gastrointestinal symptoms VAS score of the two groups before and after the treatments: A: Abdominal pain; B: Epigastric burning; C: Abdominal bloating; D: Diarrhea; E: Constipation, Table S1: Foods classification based on iron content.

Author Contributions: Conceptualization, F.B., F.F., L.E. and L.D.; Methodology, L.R. and L.E.; Investigation, A.S., F.B., F.F., and L.E.; Data Curation, K.A.B.; Formal analysis, L.R., K.A.B., and L.E.; Original Draft Preparation, A.S., L.E.; Review and Editing of Manuscript, A.S., L.R., K.A.B., and L.E.; and Funding Acquisition, M.V. All authors have read and agreed to the published version of the manuscript.

Funding: This research was funded by Fondazione IRCCS Ca' Granda and received grants from Italy's Ministry of Health and Lombardy's Regional Government Authority (Ministero della Salute e Regione Lombardia, grant number 2011-02348234). The Article Processing Charge was funded by Fondazione IRCCS Ca' Granda Ospedale Maggiore Policlinico and Università degli Studi di Milano, Milan, Italy.

Conflicts of Interest: The authors declare no conflict of interest.

References

1. Lebwohl, B.; Sanders, D.S.; Green, P.H.R. Coeliac disease. *Lancet* **2018**, *391*, 70–81. [CrossRef]

2. Van Berge-Henegouwen, G.P.; Mulder, C.J. Pioneer in the gluten free diet: Willem-Karel Dicke 1905–1962, over 50 years of gluten free diet. *Gut* **1993**, *34*, 1473–1475. [CrossRef] [PubMed]
3. Rubio-Tapia, A.; Murray, J.A. Celiac disease. *Curr. Opin. Gastroenterol.* **2010**, *26*, 116–122. [CrossRef] [PubMed]
4. Gujral, N.; Freeman, H.J.; Thomson, A.B. Celiac disease: Prevalence, diagnosis, pathogenesis and treatment. *World J. Gastroenterol.* **2012**, *18*, 6036–6059. [CrossRef]
5. Schuppan, D.; Junker, Y.; Barisani, N. Celiac Disease: From Pathogenesis to Novel Therapies. *Gastroenterology* **2009**, *137*, 1912–1933. [CrossRef]
6. Bardella, M.T.; Elli, L.; Velio, P.; Fredella, C.; Prampolini, L.; Cesana, B. Silent Celiac Disease Is Frequent in the Siblings of Newly Diagnosed Celiac Patients. *Digestion* **2007**, *75*, 182–187. [CrossRef]
7. Rubio-Tapia, A.; Hill, I.D.; Kelly, C.P.; Calderwood, A.H.; Murray, J.A. ACG Clinical Guidelines: Diagnosis and Management of Celiac Disease. *Am. J. Gastroenterol.* **2013**, *108*, 656–676. [CrossRef]
8. Ludvigsson, J.F.; Bai, J.C.; Biagi, F.; Card, T.; Ciacci, C.; Ciclitira, P.J.; Green, P.H.R.; Hadjivassiliou, M.; Holdoway, A.; Van Heel, D.A.; et al. Diagnosis and management of adult coeliac disease: Guidelines from the British Society of Gastroenterology. *Gut* **2014**, *63*, 1210–1228. [CrossRef]
9. Corazza, G.R.; Valentini, R.A.; Andreani, M.L.; D'Anchino, M.; Leva, M.T.; Ginaldi, L.; De Feudis, L.; Quaglino, D.; Gasbarrini, G. Subclinical Coeliac Disease is a Frequent Cause of Iron-Deficiency Anaemia. *Scand. J. Gastroenterol.* **1995**, *30*, 153–156. [CrossRef]
10. Carroccio, A.; Iannitto, E.; Cavataio, F.; Montalto, G.; Tumminello, M.; Campagna, P.; Lipari, M.G.; Notarbartolo, A.; Iacono, G. Sideropenic anemia and celiac disease: One study, two points of view. *Dig. Dis. Sci.* **1998**, *43*, 673–678. [CrossRef] [PubMed]
11. Annibale, B.; Severi, C.; Chistolini, A.; Antonelli, G.; Lahner, E.; Marcheggiano, A.; Iannoni, C.; Monarca, B.; Fave, G.D. Efficacy of gluten-free diet alone on recovery from iron deficiency anemia in adult celiac patients. *Am. J. Gastroenterol.* **2001**, *96*, 132–137. [CrossRef] [PubMed]
12. Halfdanarson, T.R.; Litzow, M.R.; Murray, J.A. Hematologic manifestations of celiac disease. *Blood* **2007**, *109*, 412–421. [CrossRef] [PubMed]
13. Wang, Y.; Yu, L.; Ding, J.; Chen, Y. Iron Metabolism in Cancer. *Int. J. Mol. Sci.* **2018**, *20*, 95. [CrossRef] [PubMed]
14. Dev, S.; Babitt, J.L. Overview of iron metabolism in health and disease. *Hemodial. Int.* **2017**, *21*, S6–S20. [CrossRef] [PubMed]
15. Gulec, S.; Anderson, G.J.; Collins, J.F. Mechanistic and regulatory aspects of intestinal iron absorption. *Am. J. Physiol. Gastrointest. Liver Physiol.* **2014**, *307*, G397–G409. [CrossRef] [PubMed]
16. Patterson, A.J.; Brown, W.J.; Roberts, D.C.; Seldon, M.R. Dietary treatment of iron deficiency in women of childbearing age. *Am. J. Clin. Nutr.* **2001**, *74*, 650–656. [CrossRef]
17. CREA. Centro di Ricerca Alimenti e Nutrizione—Tabelle di Composizione Degli Alimenti. Available online: https://www.crea.gov.it/alimenti-e-nutrizione (accessed on 17 October 2016).
18. Lane, D.J.; Richardson, D.R. The active role of vitamin C in mammalian iron metabolism: Much more than just enhanced iron absorption! *Free Radic. Boil. Med.* **2014**, *75*, 69–83. [CrossRef]
19. Samman, S.; Sandström, B.; Toft, M.B.; Bukhave, K.; Jensen, M.; Sørensen, S.S.; Hansen, M. Green tea or rosemary extract added to foods reduces nonheme-iron absorption. *Am. J. Clin. Nutr.* **2001**, *73*, 607–612. [CrossRef]
20. Kristensen, M.B.; Tetens, I.; Jørgensen, A.B.A.; Thomsen, A.D.; Milman, N.; Hels, O.; Sandström†, B.; Hansen, M. A decrease in iron status in young healthy women after long-term daily consumption of the recommended intake of fibre-rich wheat bread. *Eur. J. Nutr.* **2005**, *44*, 334–340. [CrossRef]
21. Centers for Disease Control and Prevention. Iron deficiency—United States, 1999–2000. *Morb. Mortal. Wkly. Rep.* **2002**, *51*, 897–899.
22. Elli, L.; Poggiali, E.; Tomba, C.; Andreozzi, F.; Nava, I.; Bardella, M.T.; Campostrini, N.; Girelli, D.; Conte, D.; Cappellini, M.D. Does TMPRSS6 RS855791 Polymorphism Contribute to Iron Deficiency in Treated Celiac Disease? *Am. J. Gastroenterol.* **2015**, *110*, 200–202. [CrossRef] [PubMed]
23. Vici, G.; Belli, L.; Biondi, M.; Polzonetti, V. Gluten free diet and nutrient deficiencies: A review. *Clin. Nutr.* **2016**, *35*, 1236–1241. [CrossRef] [PubMed]
24. Wild, D.; Robins, G.G.; Burley, V.; Howdle, P.D. Evidence of high sugar intake, and low fibre and mineral intake, in the gluten-free diet. *Aliment. Pharmacol. Ther.* **2010**, *32*, 573–581. [CrossRef]

25. Lopez, A.; Cacoub, P.; MacDougall, I.C.; Peyrin-Biroulet, L. Iron deficiency anaemia. *Lancet* **2016**, *387*, 907–916. [CrossRef]
26. Waldvogel-Abramowski, S.; Waeber, G.; Gassner, C.; Buser, A.; Frey, B.M.; Favrat, B.; Tissot, J.-D. Physiology of iron metabolism. *Transfus. Med. Hemother.* **2014**, *41*, 213–221. [CrossRef] [PubMed]
27. Tetens, I.; Bendtsen, K.M.; Henriksen, M.; Ersbøll, A.K.; Milman, N. The impact of a meat-versus a vegetable-based diet on iron status in women of childbearing age with small iron stores. *Eur. J. Nutr.* **2007**, *46*, 439–445. [CrossRef]
28. Weinborn, V.; Pizarro, F.; Olivares, M.; Brito, A.; Arredondo, M.; Flores, S.; Valenzuela, C. The Effect of Plant Proteins Derived from Cereals and Legumes on Heme Iron Absorption. *Nutrients* **2015**, *7*, 5446. [CrossRef]
29. Hurrell, R.F.; Egli, I. Iron bioavailability and dietary reference values. *Am. J. Clin. Nutr.* **2010**, *91*, 1461S–1467S. [CrossRef]
30. Hallert, C.; Grännö, C.; Grant, C.; Hultén, S.; Midhagen, G.; Ström, M.; Svensson, H.; Valdimarsson, T.; Wickström, T. Quality of life of adult coeliac patients treated for 10 years. *Scand. J. Gastroenterol.* **1998**, *33*, 933–938. [CrossRef]

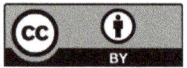

© 2020 by the authors. Licensee MDPI, Basel, Switzerland. This article is an open access article distributed under the terms and conditions of the Creative Commons Attribution (CC BY) license (http://creativecommons.org/licenses/by/4.0/).

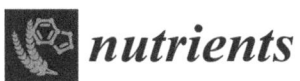

Article

Wheat Sensitivity and Functional Dyspepsia: A Pilot, Double-Blind, Randomized, Placebo-Controlled Dietary Crossover Trial with Novel Challenge Protocol

Michael D. E. Potter [1,2,3], Kerith Duncanson [1,2,*], Michael P. Jones [1,2,4], Marjorie M. Walker [1,2], Simon Keely [1,2] and Nicholas J. Talley [1,2,3]

1. Faculty of Health and Medicine, University of Newcastle, Callaghan, NSW 2308, Australia; michael.potter@newcastle.edu.au (M.D.E.P.); mike.jones@mq.edu.au (M.P.J.); marjorie.walker@newcastle.edu.au (M.M.W.); simon.keely@newcastle.edu.au (S.K.); nicholas.talley@newcastle.edu.au (N.J.T)
2. Australian Gastrointestinal Research Alliance (AGIRA), Hunter Medical Research Institute, New Lambton Heights, NSW 2305, Australia
3. Department of Gastroenterology, John Hunter Hospital, New Lambton Heights, NSW 2305, Australia
4. Psychology Department, Macquarie University, Macquarie Park, Sydney, NSW 2109, Australia
* Correspondence: kerith.duncanson@newcastle.edu.au

Received: 20 May 2020; Accepted: 27 June 2020; Published: 30 June 2020

Abstract: Introduction: Functional dyspepsia (FD), characterised by symptoms of epigastric pain or early satiety and post prandial distress, has been associated with duodenal eosinophilia, raising the possibility that it is driven by an environmental allergen. Non-coeliac gluten or wheat sensitivity (NCG/WS) has also been associated with both dyspeptic symptoms and duodenal eosinophilia, suggesting an overlap between these two conditions. The aim of this study was to evaluate the role of wheat (specifically gluten and fructans) in symptom reduction in participants with FD in a pilot randomized double-blind, placebo controlled, dietary crossover trial. Methods: Patients with Rome III criteria FD were recruited from a single tertiary centre in Newcastle, Australia. All were individually counselled on a diet low in both gluten and fermentable oligo-, di-, mono-saccharides, and polyols (FODMAPs) by a clinical dietitian, which was followed for four weeks (elimination diet phase). Those who had a ≥30% response to the run-in diet, as measured by the Nepean Dyspepsia Index, were then re-challenged with 'muesli' bars containing either gluten, fructan, or placebo in randomised order. Those with symptoms which significantly reduced during the elimination diet, but reliably reappeared (a mean change in overall dyspeptic symptoms of ≥30%) with gluten or fructan re-challenge were deemed to have wheat induced FD. Results: Eleven participants were enrolled in the study (75% female, mean age 43 years). Of the initial cohort, nine participants completed the elimination diet phase of whom four qualified for the rechallenge phase. The gluten-free, low FODMAP diet led to an overall (albeit non-significant) improvement in symptoms of functional dyspepsia in the diet elimination phase (mean NDI symptom score 71.2 vs. 47.1, $p = 0.087$). A specific food trigger could not be reliably demonstrated. Conclusions: Although a gluten-free, low-FODMAP diet led to a modest overall reduction in symptoms in this cohort of FD patients, a specific trigger could not be identified. The modified Salerno criteria for NCG/WS identification trialled in this dietary rechallenge protocol was fit-for-purpose. However, larger trials are required to determine whether particular components of wheat induce symptoms in functional dyspepsia.

Keywords: non coeliac wheat sensitivity; gluten; FODMAPs; functional dyspepsia

1. Introduction

Functional dyspepsia (FD) is a troublesome gastrointestinal disorder that affects the health and wellbeing of more than 15% of the population [1]. It is characterised by symptoms referrable to the gastroduodenal region of the abdomen, including early satiety, post-prandial fullness, and epigastric pain [2]. FD overlaps with irritable bowel syndrome (IBS) and may be mislabelled as such. Both disorders are associated with meal-related symptoms [3]. People with FD often report that certain dietary triggers exacerbate symptoms, with wheat and/or gluten commonly implicated [4]. Functional dyspepsia is also closely linked with wheat sensitivity in epidemiological studies [1].

Duodenal eosinophilia has been observed in biopsy tissue samples obtained at upper endoscopy from patients with FD, particularly in those with post-prandial distress syndrome [5–7]. In a case-control study from Sweden of 51 adults with FD, duodenal eosinophilia was significantly increased in cases compared with controls, with a mean of 33.1 and 34.6 eosinophils per five high-power fields (HPF) in FD cases in the first and second part of the duodenum (D1 and D2), compared with 18.4 and 18.6 in controls [5]. A study of 33 patients from an Australian centre replicated these observations, demonstrating duodenal (D2) eosinophilia in patients with the post-prandial distress subtype of FD [6]. Mechanistic studies have implicated duodenal eosinophils with impaired intestinal duodenal barrier and neuronal functioning [8,9], pointing towards an underlying mechanism for the disorder. An allergen (potentially wheat) or infection may lead to barrier disruption and the generation of a Th2 or Th17 type immune response, which induces recruitment and degranulation of eosinophils, affecting the submucosal nervous system and altering gastroduodenal function [10]. In the absence of a validated biomarker, it is not currently possible to attribute FD symptom generation to a specific component of wheat [11,12].

Wheat is also commonly implicated in unexplained gastrointestinal and extraintestinal symptoms termed 'non-coeliac gluten or wheat sensitivity' (NCG/WS). This disorder is characterised by wheat sensitivity (specifically self-reported adverse physiological symptoms after wheat ingestion) in the absence of demonstrable wheat allergy or coeliac disease [13,14]. Symptoms commonly reported include those which overlap with IBS, such as bloating, constipation, abdominal pain, and diarrhoea. Dyspeptic symptoms also affect more than half of those with NCWS [15] and extraintestinal symptoms are common [14]. Similar to FD, duodenal eosinophilia has been reported in NCG/WS [7]. In a group of 276 patients with NCG/WS, diagnosed by a double-blind, placebo-controlled challenge, the duodenal eosinophil count was measured to be significantly higher than both coeliac and IBS controls (63 per 10 HPF vs. 38 and 31 respectively, $p < 0.0005$) [7]. Current consensus criteria requires a blinded placebo controlled crossover challenge of gluten in order to make the diagnosis of non-coeliac gluten sensitivity (NCGS) [16].

Fructans are a type of fermentable carbohydrate common in wheat. They are implicated in IBS symptoms such as bloating and changes in bowel habit [17], but less is known about their contribution to other gastrointestinal symptoms, including dyspepsia. Wheat contributes at least 70% of total dietary fructans in the United States, averaging 2.6 g of inulin-type fructans and 2.5 g of fructo-oligosaccharide per day [18]. A food item is considered to be a substantial food sources of fructans if it contains more than 0.5 g of fructans per serving [19]. Wheat also contains amylase trypsin inhibitors (ATIs), which are non-gluten proteins capable of activating the innate immune system via interaction with toll-like receptor [14].

To better understand the relationship between wheat and symptom induction in people with FD, the effects of gluten, fructan- type FODMAPs (fermentable oligo- di- mono- saccharides and polyols) and ATIs need to be differentiated. This is possible if the consensus protocol proposed for NCGS [16] is extended to account for fructans and ATIs. The Salerno Experts' Criteria for diagnosis of NCGS (2015) recommends a double-blind, randomised crossover trial that provides at least eight grams of gluten (cooked into food, not capsule) a day in the gluten challenge phase. This dose approximates the average daily intake of gluten in Western countries (10–15 g) [20]. Adding a wheat fructan dietary challenge arm to the Salerno criteria protocol would mean the role of gluten and fructans could be differentiated. A daily dose of fructans of at least 2.5 g would be expected to induce symptoms in those with fructan sensitivity, but not in the general population.

The primary aim of the current study was to ascertain whether a wheat free diet, specifically a gluten-free and low-FODMAP diet, induced a significant reduction in symptoms in patients with functional dyspepsia. Our secondary aim was to demonstrate whether gluten or fructans were responsible for the improvement in those who responded to the wheat free diet, using a placebo-controlled, blinded re-challenge. We also tested a novel double-blind, randomised crossover trial design for gluten and fructan challenges to differentiate potential wheat components implicated in FD symptom induction.

2. Methods

2.1. Participants

Adult participants (age 8–80 years) were recruited from the outpatient gastroenterology clinics at John Hunter Hospital, a tertiary referral centre located on the mid-north coast of New South Wales, Australia (Figure S1). Participants fulfilled Rome III criteria for functional dyspepsia based on symptoms and a negative upper endoscopy [20]. All participants tested negative for coeliac disease (with negative anti-tissue transglutaminase IgA and normal duodenal biopsies) and wheat allergy (negative wheat specific serum IgE). Those with inflammatory bowel disease, active malignancy or infection, and pregnant patients were excluded.

2.2. Protocol

The study design was modified from the Salerno criteria, the currently accepted standard for the diagnosis of NCG/WS [16]. Participants, ideally on a normal wheat-containing diet for 4 weeks, completed a food frequency questionnaire [21], and were instructed on a low-FODMAP, gluten-free diet by a clinical dietitian (Figure 1).

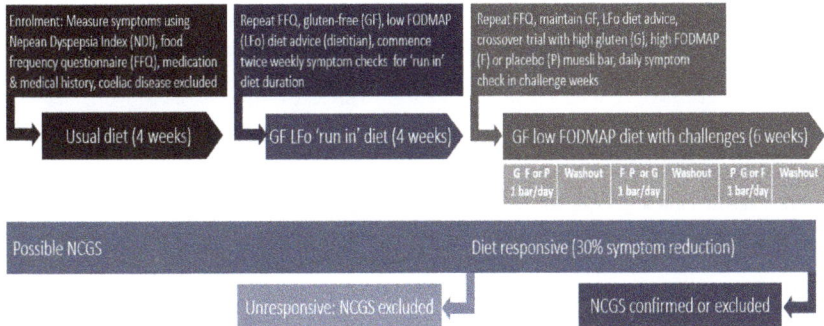

Figure 1. Non coeliac gluten/wheat sensitivity protocol overview including: 'Run in phase' (dark grey); baseline clinical testing, baseline diet assessment; gluten-free, low-fermentable oligo-, di-, mono-saccharides, and polyols (FODMAP) diet instruction by dietitian, four-week 'run-in' diet phase with pre-post symptom measurement, and second-daily dyspeptic symptom measurement; 'Dietary challenge phase' (dark blue); gluten-free, low-FODMAP diet continued, one challenge bar per day for one week (order of bars randomized) with high gluten, high fructan/FODMAP and placebo bars, with symptoms measured daily using a visual, analogue scale. Key: GF: Gluten free; FODMAP: Fermentable oligo- di- mono- saccharides and polyols; NCGS: Non-coeliac gluten sensitivity.

Symptoms were assessed at baseline and after 4 weeks using the validated Nepean Dyspepsia Index (NDI) [22]. A food frequency questionnaire was used to calculate the change (mean, grams per day) in FODMAP intake over the run-in diet period [21], and a validated questionnaire was used to ensure compliance with the gluten-free aspect of the diet [23] (Figure S2). Those with a significant reduction in symptoms after the run-in diet (defined as ≥30% reduction in NDI score) were eligible for the rechallenge phase. This involved continuation of the low-FODMAP, gluten-free baseline diet with the addition of one 'challenge' bar per day (to replace a snack) for one week at a time, separated by a week-long washout period. The order in which the three 'challenge' bars were consumed by participants was randomized using a computer generated randomization algorithm, with the bar order contained in written instructions that were stored in a sealed envelope and given to each participant at the beginning of the re-challenge phase, blinding the research assistant to treatment allocation. Participants were assigned bars containing fructans (approximately 6.9 g inulin, without gluten), gluten (approximately 8.5 g gluten [24], with low fructan content), and placebo (without fructans or other FODMAPs, gluten-free ingredients) (Supplementary Files 1 and 2). The bars were independently tested for FODMAP content by an external laboratory prior to trial commencement (FODMAP friendly, Pty Ltd., Victoria, Australia) to confirm FODMAP content. All bars were nutritionally equivalent and indistinguishable in look, texture, and taste (Figure 2) but labelled as Bar A, Bar B, or Bar C to align with double-blinded randomization process.

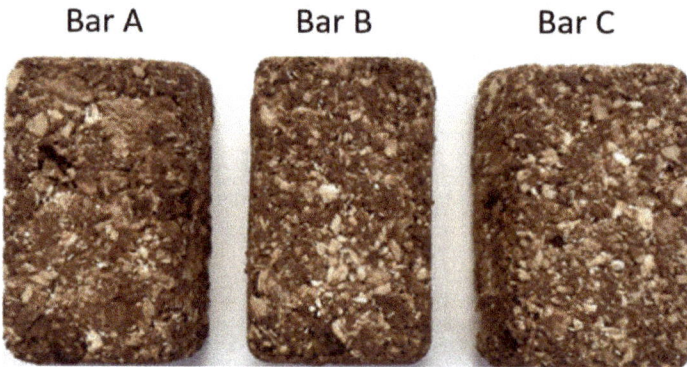

Figure 2. Three visually indistinguishable, nutritionally equivalent 'muesli' bars with differing gluten and fructan contents used for a functional dyspepsia randomized, double-blind crossover trial.

Dyspeptic symptoms were measured daily during the rechallenge phase and weekly during the washout weeks using a numbered visual analogue scale (VAS) (3 main symptoms; post-prandial fullness, epigastric pain, early satiety, each scored 0–10) [16].

This study received Hunter New England Human Research Ethics Committee approval on March 18, 2018 (ethics approval number: 2019/ETH01181). The study is registered as Australia New Zealand Clinical Trial: ID Number: 380018.

2.3. Sample Size and Statistics

Our sample size calculation was based on the hypothesis that a dietary trigger is responsible for symptoms with FD, and that the dietary response would be due to gluten or FODMAP intake. Using repeated measures analysis of variance, with a power of 0.8 and a significance of 0.025 (0.05/2 for dual hypothesis) and a delta of 0.5, we calculated that we required 41 subjects to enter the dietary challenge phase of the trial. Assuming that 30% of subjects would not respond to the run-in diet and be eliminated, we estimated 58 participants would need to commence the study. Statistical analysis was performed using STATA software (StataCorp, TX, USA).

Changes in FODMAP intake and symptoms between run-in and diet phase were evaluated via repeated measures analysis of variance. Association between baseline factors and change in symptoms was evaluated via linear regression.

3. Results

Eleven participants were enrolled in the study between July 2018 and February 2019 (75% female, mean age 43 years). Regarding the functional dyspepsia subtype, four had epigastric pain syndrome, two had postprandial distress, and five fulfilled criteria for both (overlap syndrome). Four participants were already following a partial exclusionary diet (three partially avoiding gluten and/or FODMAPs, one following a low FODMAP diet). The sample size of 41 participants was not achieved in the study timeframe due to logistical reasons.

After the run-in diet, the mean FODMAP intake decreased from 40.1 g to 17.1 g ($p = 0.14$) (Figure 3 and Figure S3), and all were adherent to gluten exclusion based on the applied questionnaire [23].

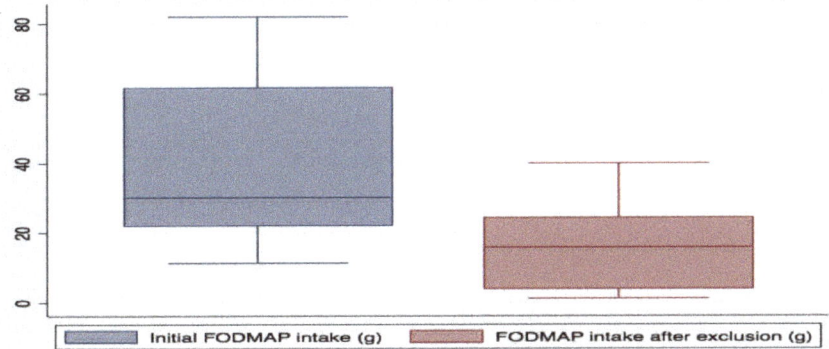

Figure 3. Total FODMAP (fermentable oligo-, di-, and monosaccharides, and polyols, gram per day) intake before (n = 8) and after (n = 5) commencement of low-FODMAP, gluten-free diet, as measured by the food frequency questionnaire ($p = 0.14$, Wilcoxon signed-rank test).

Of the initial 11 participant cohort, nine completed the run-in diet phase. The gluten-free, low-FODMAP run-in diet led to an overall improvement in symptoms of functional dyspepsia (mean NDI symptom score 71.2 vs. 47.1, $p = 0.087$; Figure 4 and Figure S4).

There was no significant association between the baseline eosinophil count and the magnitude of change in dyspeptic symptoms during the run-in diet period ($p = 0.45$, linear regression, Figure 5). Two participants reported worsening of constipation symptoms, and one worsening of bloating and constipation requiring cessation of the run-in diet.

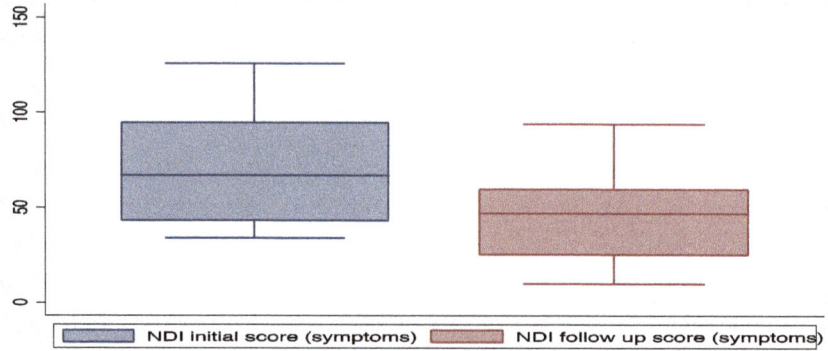

Figure 4. Mean symptom scores before (n = 10) and after (n = 8) the gluten-free, low-FODMAP diet (p = 0.087, Wilcoxon sign rank test). NDI—Nepean dyspepsia index.

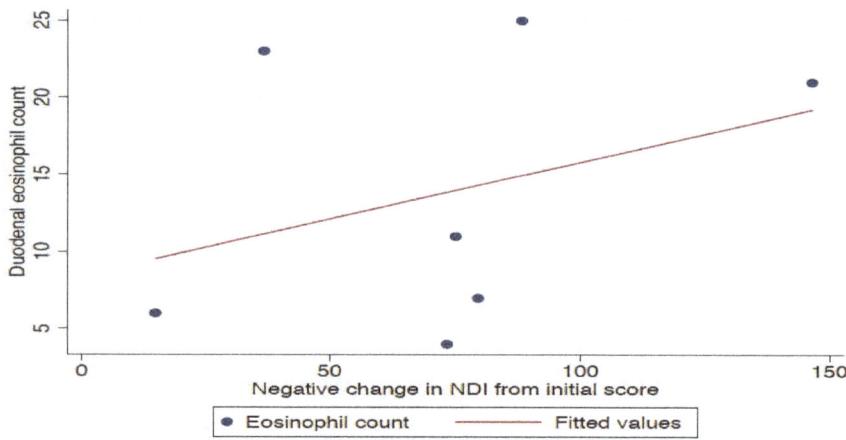

Figure 5. Relationship between duodenal eosinophil count and magnitude of change in the severity of dyspeptic symptoms measured with the Nepean Dyspepsia Index (NDI) after the run-in diet (p = 0.45, r^2 = 0.12). Duodenal eosinophil count expressed per mm^2. Four subjects qualified for the rechallenge phase, based on a >30% reduction in their NDI score. Three out of four of these participants completed the protocol. Meaningful analysis of the data was not possible, however there was no signal that one bar caused symptom worsening compared to other bars.

4. Discussion

An overall reduction in dyspeptic symptoms was observed with removal of wheat gluten and fructans, but the association was not significant. Therefore, we have not demonstrated a link between FD and NCG/WS. Early termination of the study due to under-recruitment and low eligibility for the challenge phase resulted in the dietary re-challenge not being conducted by a meaningful number of participants.

Our study demonstrated a trend towards improvement in dyspeptic symptoms on a wheat-free, low-FODMAP diet. The mean total FODMAP intake reported at baseline in this FD cohort was higher than total FODMAP intake of IBS sufferers who had returned to a 'habitual' diet (40.1 versus 29.4 g per day) in a study on long-term outcomes of a FODMAP-modified diet, using the same dietary assessment tool [25]. The post 'run-in' FODMAP intake in our study approximated the intake of those who continued on a FODMAP restricted diet in the same long-term outcome study (17.1 versus 20.6 g per day) [25]. Despite the low participant numbers at both baseline (n = 8) and post 'run in' (n = 5), these results indicate that a low FODMAP intake was achieved in the 'run-in' phase by this FD cohort.

After four weeks of a gluten-free diet and 57% reduced mean FODMAPs intake (grams per day), participants (n = 9) reported a 33% reduction in FD symptom score. This is consistent with previous observational studies [4] and one intervention study [26] that demonstrated a link between wheat-based foods and symptoms in people with functional dyspepsia. Elli et al. [26] recruited 134 participants with a Rome III diagnosis of FD and IBS. Seventy-five percent (n = 98) reported improvement in symptoms on an initial GFD and progressed to the blinded trial phase. Of this participant subset, 14% (10% of original study sample) reported recurrence of symptoms with blinded gluten capsule challenges, fulfilling a clinical diagnosis of NCG/WS. Two out of four specific symptoms that showed a significant association with gluten ingestion in the blinded challenge are associated with FD rather than IBS (post prandial fullness ($p = 0.01$), and early satiety ($p = 0.03$)) [26].

We did not demonstrate an association between the number of duodenal eosinophils at baseline and the subsequent symptom response, although given the small numbers of participants recruited this may be due to under-powering. Further studies with a sample size of at least 50 participants are needed to establish whether duodenal eosinophilia may be a biomarker for wheat sensitive FD.

4.1. Limitations

Only 11 participants enrolled in this trial from an expected sample size of approximately 60 people. It is possible that the dietary requirements of the trial were prohibitive for prospective participants, or that the study needed a longer recruitment period or more study sites. Twenty-seven percent (n = 3/11) of participants completed the 14-week study. This high attrition rate was partly attributable to participants being ineligible to proceed into the crossover trial if they did not achieve a > 30% reduction in their NDI score. In future studies, our study criteria will be revised to account for, but not exclude based on symptom reduction.

As participants who experienced exacerbation of symptoms did not complete the post run-in diet FFQ, it is not known whether they had reduced FODMAP intake, or if other lifestyle factors, such as stress, influenced symptom induction. The study was under-powered to demonstrate an association between the number of duodenal eosinophils at baseline and the subsequent symptom response after the 'run-in' diet. It was also under-powered to detect a signal that one type of bar caused symptom worsening compared to the other two bars. Finally, ATIs from wheat have been shown to activate TLR4, triggering innate immune effects and increasing low level inflammation [14]. ATIs were not measured in this study but should be considered in future studies that aim to distinguish between respective wheat components in NCG/WS and FD.

Following a gluten-free, low-FODMAP diet is expensive and difficult to maintain, even if the individual receives advice and support from a dietitian and experiences a reduction in symptoms. We recommend that future studies involve the provision of some low FODMAP, gluten-free grocery items to reduce the financial burden, and to increase participant retention and dietary compliance.

4.2. Implication for Practice and Research

Despite this study being underpowered to detect an association between wheat component intake and FD symptom induction, there are some implications for clinicians and researchers.

We emphasise the importance of using Rome criteria for diagnosis of FD, and differentiation from IBS (or diagnosis of overlapping FD/IBS) as a basis for studies investigating the role of wheat and other potential symptom triggers.

Although not fully elucidated in this study, we recommend that clinicians consider the potential involvement of wheat in FD symptom induction and management. Dietitians are well positioned to support people with FD to maintain an exclusion diet that balances symptom management, diet variety, and nutritional adequacy.

We recommend that future research studies allocate funding for provision of gluten-free, low-FODMAP groceries to participants to increase recruitment, retention, and dietary compliance. We expect that assessing symptom reduction in the 'run-in' phase (without setting a strict exclusion cut-off) will increase retention into the crossover trial phase of FD and NCG/WS studies. Additional investment of research resources towards understanding the respective roles of wheat gluten, fructans, and ATIs in the intestinal and extraintestinal symptoms and characteristics of FD will substantially progress our understanding and management of functional dyspepsia.

5. Conclusions

Although a gluten-free, low-FODMAP diet led to a modest overall reduction in symptoms in this cohort of FD patients, this was not significant, and a specific trigger could not be identified using this dietary rechallenge protocol. Further larger studies are required to explore whether a wheat-free diet (either a gluten-free or low-FODMAP diet) may be of use in treating functional dyspepsia. Wheat may contribute, but even if it is a factor in FD pathogenesis, it does not seem to be solely responsible for symptoms.

6. Patents

Patented functional grain product concepts used in low-FODMAP, high-gluten muesli bar development (Australian Patent No. 2014262285; New Zealand Patent No. 629207; South Africa Patent No. 2015/07891).

Supplementary Materials: The following are available online at http://www.mdpi.com/2072-6643/12/7/1947/s1, Supplementary File 1: Modified Salerno protocol to differentiate responses to wheat gluten and/or fructans in a randomized, double-blind, placebo-controlled crossover trial. Supplementary File 2: Example Wheat Sensitivity Questionnaire: modified from The Salerno Experts' Criteria. Primary outcome: Response of dyspeptic (or NCG/WS) symptoms to dietary removal, challenge and subsequent re-challenge with gluten and FODMAPs. Secondary outcomes: Response of other gastrointestinal symptoms and extra-intestinal symptoms to dietary removal and subsequent challenge with FODMAPS and gluten.

Author Contributions: Individual author contributions to this article include: Conceptualization (M.D.E.P., S.K., M.M.W., N.J.T.); methodology (M.D.E.P., K.D., S.K., N.J.T., M.P.J.); validation (N.J.T., M.D.E.P., M.P.J.); formal analysis (M.D.E.P., M.M.W., N.J.T.); investigation (M.D.E.P., K.D.); resources (M.D.E.P., K.D.); data curation (M.D.E.P.); writing—original draft preparation (M.D.E.P.); writing—review and editing (N.J.T., S.K., M.M.W., K.D.). All authors have read and agreed to the published version of the manuscript.

Funding: This study was supported by a PhD scholarship grant to MP from the National Health & Medical Research Council and a National Health & Medical Research Council Investigator Grant (NJT).

Acknowledgments: Technical support for FODMAP testing of study trial muesli bars was provided by FODMAP Friendly, FODMAP Pty. Ltd. 1st Floor, 91 Maroondah Highway, Ringwood Victoria 3134 Australia.

Conflicts of Interest: Kerith Duncanson is a company director for the Good Gut Group, that has patented functional bread and grain product concepts (Australian Patent No. 2014262285; New Zealand Patent No. 629207; South Africa Patent No. 2015/07891) for Irritable Bowel Syndrome (IBS) consumers. Good Gut Group had no role in the design of the study; in the collection, analyses, or interpretation of data; in the writing of the manuscript, or in the decision to publish the results.

References

1. Potter, M.D.; Walker, M.M.; Jones, M.P.; Koloski, N.A.; Keely, S.; Talley, N.J. Wheat Intolerance and Chronic Gastrointestinal Symptoms in an Australian Population-based Study: Association between Wheat Sensitivity, Celiac Disease and Functional Gastrointestinal Disorders. *Am. J. Gastroenterol* **2018**, *113*, 1036–1044. [CrossRef]
2. Talley, N.J.; Ford, A.C. Functional Dyspepsia. *N. Engl. J. Med.* **2015**, *373*, 1853–1863. [CrossRef] [PubMed]
3. Von Wulffen, M.; Talley, N.J.; Hammer, J.; McMaster, J.; Rich, G.; Shah, A.; Koloski, N.; Kendall, B.J.; Jones, M.; Holtmann, G. Overlap of irritable bowel syndrome and functional dyspepsia in the clinical setting: Prevalence and risk factors. *Dig. Dis. Sci.* **2019**, *64*, 480–486. [CrossRef]
4. Duncanson, K.R.; Talley, N.J.; Walker, M.M.; Burrows, T.L. Food and functional dyspepsia: A systematic review. *J. Hum. Nutr. Diet.* **2017**, *31*, 390–407. [CrossRef]

5. Talley, N.J.; Walker, M.M.; Aro, P.; Ronkainen, J.; Storskrubb, T.; Hindley, L.A.; Harmsen, W.S.; Zinsmeister, A.R.; Agréus, L. Non-ulcer dyspepsia and duodenal eosinophilia: An adult endoscopic population-based case-control study. *Clin. Gastroenterol. Hepatol.* **2007**, *5*, 1175–1183. [CrossRef]
6. Walker, M.M.; Aggarwal, K.R.; Shim, L.S.; Bassan, M.; Kalantar, J.S.; Weltman, M.D.; Jones, M.; Powell, N.; Talley, N.J. Duodenal eosinophilia and early satiety in functional dyspepsia: Confirmation of a positive association in an Australian cohort. *J. Gastroenterol. Hepatol.* **2014**, *29*, 474–479. [CrossRef]
7. Carroccio, A.; Mansueto, P.; Iacono, G.; Soresi, M.; D'alcamo, A.; Cavataio, F.; Brusca, I.; Florena, A.M.; Ambrosiano, G.; Seidita, A.; et al. Non-celiac wheat sensitivity diagnosed by double-blind placebo-controlled challenge: Exploring a new clinical entity. *Am. J. Gastroenterol.* **2012**, *107*, 1898–1906. [CrossRef]
8. Vanheel, H.; Vicario, M.; Vanuytsel, T.; Van Oudenhove, L.; Martinez, C.; Keita, Å.V.; Pardon, N.; Santos, J.; Söderholm, J.D.; Tack, J.; et al. Impaired duodenal mucosal integrity and low-grade inflammation in functional dyspepsia. *Gut* **2014**, *63*, 262–271. [CrossRef]
9. Cirillo, C.; Bessissow, T.; Desmet, A.S.; Vanheel, H.; Tack, J.; Berghe, P.V. Evidence for neuronal and structural changes in submucous ganglia of patients with functional dyspepsia. *Am. J. Gastroenterol.* **2015**, *110*, 1205–1215. [CrossRef] [PubMed]
10. Talley, N.J. What causes functional gastrointestinal disorders? A proposed disease model. *Am. J. Gastroenterol.* **2020**, *115*, 41–48. [CrossRef]
11. Biesiekierski, J.R.; Peters, S.L.; Newnham, E.D.; Rosella, O.; Muir, J.G.; Gibson, P.R. No effects of gluten in patients with self-reported non-celiac gluten sensitivity after dietary reduction of fermentable, poorly absorbed, short-chain carbohydrates. *Gastroenterology* **2013**, *145*, 320–328. [CrossRef]
12. Junker, Y.; Zeissig, S.; Kim, S.J.; Barisani, D.; Wieser, H.; Leffler, D.A.; Zevallos, V.; Libermann, T.A.; Dillon, S.; Freitag, T.L.; et al. Wheat amylase trypsin inhibitors drive intestinal inflammation via activation of toll-like receptor 4. *J. Exp. Med.* **2012**, *209*, 2395–2408. [CrossRef]
13. Potter, M.D.E.; Walker, M.M.; Talley, N.J. Non-coeliac gluten or wheat sensitivity: Emerging disease or misdiagnosis? *Med. J. Aust.* **2017**, *207*, 211–215. [CrossRef]
14. Zevallos, V.F.; Raker, V.; Tenzer, S.; Jimenez-Calvente, C.; Ashfaq-Khan, M.; Rüssel, N.; Pickert, G.; Schild, H.; Steinbrink, K.; Schuppan, D. Nutritional wheat amylase-trypsin inhibitors promote intestinal inflammation via activation of myeloid cells. *Gastroenterology* **2017**, *152*, 1100–1113. [CrossRef] [PubMed]
15. Volta, U.; Bardella, M.T.; Calabrò, A.; Troncone, R.; Corazza, G.R. An Italian prospective multicenter survey on patients suspected of having non-celiac gluten sensitivity. *BMC Med.* **2014**, *12*, 85. [CrossRef]
16. Catassi, C.; Elli, L.; Bonaz, B.; Bouma, G.; Carroccio, A.; Castillejo, G.; Cellier, C.; Cristofori, F.; De Magistris, L.; Dolinsek, J.; et al. Diagnosis of Non-Celiac Gluten Sensitivity (NCGS): The Salerno Experts' Criteria. *Nutrients* **2015**, *7*, 4966–4977. [CrossRef]
17. Skodje, G.I.; Sarna, V.K.; Minelle, I.H.; Rolfsen, K.L.; Muir, J.G.; Gibson, P.R.; Veierød, M.B.; Henriksen, C.; Lundin, K.E. Fructan, Rather than Gluten, Induces Symptoms in Patients with Self-reported Non-celiac Gluten Sensitivity. *Gastroenterology* **2017**, *154*, 529–539. [CrossRef]
18. Moshfegh, A.J.; Friday, J.E.; Goldman, J.P.; Ahuja, J.K. Presence of inulin and oligofructose in the diets of Americans. *J. Nutr.* **1999**, *129*, 1407S–1411S. [CrossRef]
19. Shepherd, S.J.; Gibson, P.R. Fructose malabsorption and symptoms of irritable bowel syndrome: Guidelines for effective dietary management. *J. Am. Diet. Assoc.* **2006**, *106*, 1631–1639. [CrossRef]
20. Whitehead, W.E.; Palsson, O.; Thiwan, S.M.; Talley, N.J.; Chey, W.; Irvine, E.J.; Drossman, D.A.; Thompson, W.G.; Walker, L. *Development and Validation of the Rome III Diagnostic Questionnaire. Rome III: The Functional Gastrointestinal Disorders*, 3rd ed.; Degnon Associates, Inc.: McLean, VA, USA, 2006.
21. Barrett, J.S.; Gibson, P.R. Development and validation of a comprehensive semi-quantitative food frequency questionnaire that includes FODMAP intake and glycemic index. *J. Am. Diet. Assoc.* **2010**, *110*, 1469–1476. [CrossRef]
22. Talley, N.J.; Haque, M.; Wyeth, J.W.; Stace, N.H.; Tytgat, G.N.; Stanghellini, V.; Holtmann, G.; Verlinden, M.; Jones, M. Development of a new dyspepsia impact scale: The Nepean Dyspepsia Index. *Aliment Pharm. Ther.* **1999**, *13*, 225–235. [CrossRef] [PubMed]
23. Biagi, F.; Bianchi, P.I.; Marchese, A.; Trotta, L.; Vattiato, C.; Balduzzi, D.; Brusco, G.; Andrealli, A.; Cisaro, F.; Astegiano, M.; et al. A score that verifies adherence to a gluten-free diet: A cross-sectional, multicentre validation in real clinical life. *Br. J. Nutr.* **2012**, *108*, 1884–1888. [CrossRef] [PubMed]

24. Assor, E.; Davies-Shaw, J.; Marcon, A.; Mahmud, H. Estimation of dietary gluten content using total protein in relation to gold standard testing in a variety of foods. *J. Nutr. Food Sci.* **2014**, *4*, 1. [CrossRef]
25. O'keeffe, M.; Jansen, C.; Martin, L.; Williams, M.; Seamark, L.; Staudacher, H.M.; Irving, P.M.; Whelan, K.; Lomer, M.C. Long-term impact of the low-FODMAP diet on gastrointestinal symptoms, dietary intake, patient acceptability, and healthcare utilization in irritable bowel syndrome. *Neurogastroenterol. Motil.* **2018**, *30*, e13154. [CrossRef] [PubMed]
26. Elli, L.; Tomba, C.; Branchi, F.; Roncoroni, L.; Lombardo, V.; Bardella, M.T.; Ferretti, F.; Conte, D.; Valiante, F.; Fini, L.; et al. Evidence for the Presence of Non-Celiac Gluten Sensitivity in Patients with Functional Gastrointestinal Symptoms: Results from a Multicenter Randomized Double-Blind Placebo-Controlled Gluten Challenge. *Nutrients* **2016**, *8*, 84. [CrossRef] [PubMed]

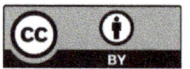

© 2020 by the authors. Licensee MDPI, Basel, Switzerland. This article is an open access article distributed under the terms and conditions of the Creative Commons Attribution (CC BY) license (http://creativecommons.org/licenses/by/4.0/).

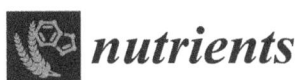

Article

Wheat Consumption Leads to Immune Activation and Symptom Worsening in Patients with Familial Mediterranean Fever: A Pilot Randomized Trial

Antonio Carroccio [1,*], Pasquale Mansueto [1], Maurizio Soresi [1], Francesca Fayer [1], Diana Di Liberto [2], Erika Monguzzi [3], Marianna Lo Pizzo [2], Francesco La Blasca [1], Girolamo Geraci [4], Alice Pecoraro [5], Francesco Dieli [2,6] and Detlef Schuppan [3,7,*]

[1] Department of Health Promotion Sciences, Maternal and Infant Care, Internal Medicine and Medical Specialties (PROMISE), University of Palermo, 90124 Palermo, Italy; pasquale.mansueto@unipa.it (P.M.); maurizio.soresi@unipa.it (M.S.); francesca.fayer@gmail.com (F.F.); francescolablasca@gmail.com (F.L.B.)
[2] Central Laboratory of Advanced Diagnosis and Biomedical Research (CLADIBIOR), University of Palermo, 90129 Palermo, Italy; diana.diliberto@unipa.it (D.D.L.); lopizzomarianna@gmail.com (M.L.P.); francesco.dieli@unipa.it (F.D.)
[3] Institute of Translational Immunology and Research Center for Immunotherapy, University Medical Center, Johannes Gutenberg University, 55122 Mainz, Germany; erika.monguzzi@gmail.com
[4] Surgery Department, University of Palermo, 90129 Palermo, Italy; girolamo.geraci@unipa.it
[5] Hematology Unit for Rare Diseases, Laboratory of Molecular Genetic, Villa Sofia-Cervello, 90146 Palermo, Italy; a.pecoraro@villasofia.it
[6] Department of Biomedicine, Neurosciences and Advanced Diagnostics (BIND), University of Palermo, 90129 Palermo, Italy
[7] Division of Gastroenterology, Beth Israel Deaconess Medical Center, Harvard Medical School, Boston, MA 02215, USA
[*] Correspondence: acarroccio@hotmail.com (A.C.); detlefschuppan@yahoo.com (D.S.); Fax: +39-091-6552884 (A.C. & D.S.)

Received: 12 February 2020; Accepted: 15 April 2020; Published: 17 April 2020

Abstract: We have identified a clinical association between self-reported non-celiac wheat sensitivity (NCWS) and Familial Mediterranean Fever (FMF). Objectives: A) To determine whether a 2-week double-blind placebo-controlled (DBPC) cross-over wheat vs. rice challenge exacerbates the clinical manifestations of FMF; B) to evaluate innate immune responses in NCWS/FMF patients challenged with wheat vs. rice. The study was conducted at the Department of Internal Medicine of the University Hospital of Palermo and the Hospital of Sciacca, Italy. Six female volunteers with FMF/NCWS (mean age 36 ± 6 years) were enrolled, 12 age-matched non-FMF, NCWS females, and 8 sex- and age-matched healthy subjects served as controls. We evaluated: 1. clinical symptoms by the FMF-specific AIDAI (Auto-Inflammatory Diseases Activity Index) score; 2. serum soluble CD14 (sCD14), C-reactive protein (CRP), and serum amyloid A (SSA); 3. circulating $CD14^+$ monocytes expressing interleukin (IL)-1β and tumor necrosis factor (TNF)-α. The AIDAI score significantly increased in FMF patients during DBPC with wheat, but not with rice (19 ± 6.3 vs. 7 ± 1.6; $p = 0.028$). sCD14 values did not differ in FMF patients before and after the challenge, but were higher in FMF patients than in healthy controls (median values 11357 vs. 8710 pg/ml; $p = 0.002$). The percentage of circulating $CD14^+/IL-1\beta^+$ and of $CD14^+/TNF-\alpha^+$ monocytes increased significantly after DBPC with wheat vs. baseline or rice challenge. Self-reported NCWS can hide an FMF diagnosis. Wheat ingestion exacerbated clinical and immunological features of FMF. Future studies performed on consecutive FMF patients recruited in centers for auto-inflammatory diseases will determine the real frequency and relevance of this association.

Keywords: AIDAI score; amylase trypsin inhibitor; non-celiac wheat sensitivity; CD14 lymphocytes; interleukin-1beta; tumor necrosis factor-α

1. Introduction

Non-celiac wheat sensitivity (NCWS) is defined as a condition of self-reported symptoms after ingestion of wheat or other gluten-containing foods, after exclusion of celiac disease (CeD), and IgE-mediated wheat allergy [1]. NCWS is characterized by intestinal or extra-intestinal symptoms, such as fatigue, headache, or joint pain that improve on a wheat (gluten)-free diet [2]. The diagnosis is established when symptoms re-occur after exposure to wheat in a double-blind placebo-controlled (DBPC) challenge [3]. Its pathogenesis, although still debated, appears to be based on a prevalent activation of the innate immune system [4].

Familial Mediterranean fever (FMF) is an auto-inflammatory disease, due to an autosomal recessive mutation in the pyrin gene. This predisposes patients to unpredictable attacks of abdominal pain, fever, and malaise, caused by serositis, mainly peritonitis and pleuritis. FMF usually manifests as short and irregular attacks which spontaneously resolve within 2–3 days. Abdominal pain and fever are the most frequent symptom of FMF. Small bowel mucosal damage has been demonstrated by capsule endoscopy in 50% of FMF patients [5]. Therefore, FMF patients are frequently first seen by gastroenterologists in search for a diagnosis. Besides the above-mentioned genetic basis of FMF, emotional stress, viral disease, or menstruation can trigger bouts of the disease. FMF pathogenesis is linked to an overshooting generalized innate immune response that is dominated by interleukin-1β (IL-1β) and tumor necrosis factor-α (TNF-α), and characterized by a generalized serositis [6]. Current treatment of choice is regular oral colchicine that suppresses excessive monocyte activation [7].

In the past years, we observed an association between NCWS and FMF. Patients with self-reported symptoms due to wheat ingestion who came to our attention had a final diagnosis of FMF associated to NCWS (FMF/NCWS).

In this pilot study, 6 patients with FMF/NCWS were subjected to a DBPC wheat vs. rice challenge, A) to assess clinical disease activity; and B) to study circulating and serum markers of systemic (innate) immune activation, compared to other patients with NCWS and healthy controls (HC). These limited data might represent a rationale for future definitive trials to assess the real prevalence of wheat-related symptoms and the putative role of wheat-free diet in FMF patients.

2. Materials and Methods

2.1. Patients

Between January 2015 and December 2017, a total of 22 patients received a new FMF diagnosis according to the Tel Hashomer Medical Center criteria [8] at the Department of Internal Medicine of the University Hospital of Palermo and of the Hospital of Sciacca, Italy.

Fifteen of them self-reported symptoms due to wheat ingestion (68%), whereas 7 did not report symptom exacerbation related to wheat (Figure 1).

Of the 15 patients reporting symptoms on wheat ingestion, 2 patients received a definitive diagnosis of CeD and 5 had a negative DBPC wheat challenge. The remaining 8 FMF patients (36% of the whole FMF group) were confirmed as FMF/NCWS patients by the DBPC wheat challenge. Of these, 6 accepted to enroll in this study (all females, mean age 36 ± 6 years), whereas 2 patients refused, as they did not accept a re-exposure to wheat ingestion. The 6 FMF patients included were on a wheat-free diet for 12–48 months (median 18) before enrollment and accepted to undergo a second DBPC wheat challenge between January and June 2019.

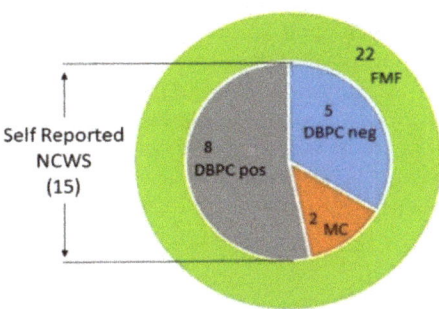

Figure 1. Number of self-reported non-celiac wheat sensitivity (NCWS) patients and of patients diagnosed with a "gluten-related" disease (celiac disease or NCWS), among 22 consecutive patients diagnosed with Familial Mediterranean Fever (FMF) in the 2 centers involved in the study. DBPC= double blind placebo-controlled challenge.

Exclusion criteria were: (a) age <18 years; (b) refusal to reintroduce wheat in the diet; (c) corticosteroids or non-steroidal anti-inflammatory drugs in the 2 weeks before biologic sample collection (blood and rectal mucosal biopsies); (d) presence of other "organic" gastrointestinal diseases; (e) pregnancy; (f) infectious diseases.

Two different control groups were recruited in the same centers. The first was composed of 12 patients (all females, mean age 35 ± 9 years), confirmed as NCWS by means of DBPC wheat challenge, who were not affected by FMF and/or other gastrointestinal diseases. They served to evaluate how far there may be differences in the inflammatory monocyte/cytokine patterns between NCWS subjects in a symptomatic phase (when they were consuming a wheat-containing diet) and the FMF/NCWS patients on the wheat challenge. They were chosen at random from patients who were enrolled in other studies on NCWS. All were matched to the FMF patients for sex and age. These subjects were symptomatic (mainly abdominal symptoms, resembling irritable bowel syndrome) on the DBPC wheat challenge. Eight healthy subjects HC, who underwent colonoscopy for colon carcinoma screening, as first-degree relatives were affected, served as additional sex- and age-matched controls. Clinical characteristics of FMF/NCWS patients are given in Supplemental file 1 (Table S1).

2.2. Methods

NCWS was diagnosed as previously described [9], with patients meeting the proposed criteria [1]. Other gastrointestinal diseases, in particular CeD, inflammatory bowel disease (IBD), and IgE-mediated wheat allergy, were carefully excluded as follows.

Exclusion of CeD:

Before evaluation for NCWS, patients were instructed to eat foods containing wheat, consuming the equivalent of at least 5 slices of wheat bread per day (about 12 grams of gluten) for 4 weeks. At the end of this period, all patients underwent serum testing for antibodies to tissue transglutaminase (anti-tTG) IgA, antibodies to deamidated gliadin peptides (anti-DGP) IgG, and antibodies to gliadin (AGA) IgA and IgG, as measured using commercial kits (Eu-tTG IgA, and anti-gliadin IgA and IgG, Eurospital Pharma, Trieste, Italy; Quanta-Lite Gliadin IgG II, Inova Diagnostics, San Diego, CA, USA). Patients were also typed for HLA-DQ2/8 phenotypes by polymerase chain reaction, using sequence-specific primers with a rapid detection method (DQ-CD Typing Plus kit by BioDiaGene, Palermo, Italy). Patients positive for the DQ2 and/or the DQ8 haplotypes also underwent duodenal mucosal biopsy, regardless of the results of the CeD-specific antibody assay.

CeD diagnosis was excluded when: A) DQ2 and/or DQ8 haplotypes were absent, or B) anti-tTG IgA and anti-DPG IgG were negative and duodenal histology showed a normal villus/crypt ratio (≥3).

Furthermore, CeD diagnosis was considered likely if patients were positive for anti-endomysial antibodies (EmA) in the medium of cultured duodenal biopsies, even if the villus/crypt ratio in the duodenal mucosa was normal. Consequently, these patients were not included in the NCWS group.

Exclusion of IBD:

IBD diagnosis was excluded when serum C-reactive protein (CRP), erythrocyte sedimentation rate, and white blood cell count were normal in repeated examinations, performed when the patients were symptomatic. Furthermore, all patients underwent abdominal ultrasound evaluation of the intestine, and those with ultrasound signs of suspected IBD were excluded. Patients with a clinical history of suspected IBD (i.e., presence of rectal bleeding or hematochezia) also underwent a complete ileo-colonoscopy. IBD diagnosis was excluded in those whose endoscopy and histology were negative.

Exclusion of IgE-mediated wheat allergy:

IgE-mediated wheat allergy was excluded by negative IgE-serum titers for wheat and/or negative skin prick test for wheat.

Elimination diet and DBPC food challenge for NCWS diagnosis:

After exclusion of CeD, IBD, IgE-mediated wheat allergy, and other gastrointestinal diseases, the patients underwent the DBPC wheat challenge for NCWS diagnosis, according to our established protocol [9]. In brief, before final NCWS diagnosis, all patients were on a standard elimination diet, which excluded wheat, cow's milk, eggs, tomato, and chocolate. Patients with self-reported food hypersensitivity excluded ingestion also of other food(s) causing symptoms. Food diaries were kept during the elimination diet, to assess dietary intake and adherence to the diet.

After 4 weeks of the elimination diet, DBPC challenges were performed according to a computer-generated sequence determined by an observer not involved in the study. For confirmation of NCWS, patients received sachets, coded A or B, containing 80 g of wheat or rice flour, respectively. Sachets A or B were given once daily, at dinner, for 2 consecutive weeks, and then after 1 week of washout, patients received the other sachets for another 2 weeks (cross-over design). If needed, the washout period was, eventually, extended for a maximum of another 2 weeks, until the symptoms induced by the previous challenge had completely resolved, before starting the next challenge.

Wheat or rice flour, given in sachets, was consumed after cooking, as determined by the patients themselves, and there was no overt difference in their appearance. Physicians assessing outcomes (AC, PM, FLB, MS) were blinded in respect to the flours ingested (wheat or rice). Wheat sachets contained 6.5 g of gluten and an estimated 0.3 g of amylase trypsin inhibitors (ATIs), as determined by bioassay [10]. The codes of the sachets were broken only at the end of the study, and the investigators did not know their contents during the study period. Challenges for other foods in patients with suspected multiple food hypersensitivities were performed in an open fashion.

During all phases of the evaluation, the severity of symptoms was recorded: patients completed a 10 point visual analog scale (VAS, with 0 representing no and 10 intolerable symptoms), which assessed the following overall symptoms and the following specific symptoms: abdominal pain or discomfort, abdominal distension, bloating, increased flatus, diarrhea (increased passage and/or urgent need for defecation of loose stools), constipation (decreased passage of stools or feeling of incomplete evacuation), heartburn, acid regurgitation, nausea and vomiting. Extra-intestinal symptoms were also recorded: rash/dermatitis, headache, foggy mind, fatigue, fainting, numbness of the limbs, joint/muscle pains, oral/tongue lesions, or other specific symptoms reported by the individual patient.

The challenges were stopped when severe clinical reactions occurred for at least 2 consecutive days (increase in VAS score >30% over the basal value) for intestinal and/or extra-intestinal symptoms. Challenges were considered positive and NCWS confirmed when the same symptoms that had been initially present initially, reappeared, after their disappearance on the elimination diet, on the wheat flour challenge and when the VAS score was >30% over the basal values.

DBPC wheat challenge performed in the present study:

The challenge protocol used for the present study was almost identical to that described above for establishing the diagnosis of NCWS. At study entry, all patients were on a wheat-free diet.

Randomization and DBPC wheat vs. rice flour challenge were performed as described above. The symptoms for the Auto-Inflammatory Disease Activity Index (AIDAI) score were recorded by the patients themselves on the scoring sheet; clinical reactions were also evaluated by 4 of the authors (AC, PM, FLB, MS).

FMF clinical evaluation:

A modified version of the AIDAI was used to assess disease activity in FMF [11]. AIDAI is a validated instrument designed to standardize the assessment of FMF clinical activity and to objectivate the FMF patients' symptoms' change across trials. In its current form, the AIDAI score is very easy to use by the patients themselves.

The ADAI score was calculated daily during the 2 weeks before the beginning of the challenge and during the periods of the DBPC challenge (2 weeks on wheat challenge and 2 weeks on placebo). AIDAI consists of 12 items: fever, overall symptoms, abdominal pain, nausea/vomiting, diarrhea, headaches, chest pain, painful nodes, arthralgia or myalgia, swelling of the joints, eye manifestations, skin rash. It was scored as yes (1 point) or no (0 point); therefore, the sum score on a single day can range between 0 to 12, and in the 14-day period, from 0 to 168 (see Supplemental file 2).

Blood sampling:

In FMF patients, venous blood samples were obtained immediately before the challenge. Additional blood samples were collected at the end of the two challenge periods.

Blood samples of NCWS patients were obtained when they were symptomatic, on a wheat-containing diet, and from HC.

Markers of inflammation:

The following serum parameters were determined by commercial ELISAs: soluble CD14 (sCD14) (R&D Systems), CRP (Roche Diagnostics S.p.A, Italia), and serum amyloid A (SAA).

Isolation of peripheral blood mononuclear cells and flow cytometry analysis:

Peripheral blood mononuclear cell (PBMC) were isolated from heparinized blood by Ficoll-Hypaque (Sigma) density-gradient centrifugation (2000 rpm for 20 min). For gating strategy see Supplemental file 3.

2.3. Statistical Analysis

Sample size was not calculated since it was a pilot study including a few number of patients. Gaussian values were expressed as mean ± SD. For parameters with non-Gaussian distribution, values were expressed as range and median. Differences between the groups were calculated using the Kruskall–Wallis test, applying the Mann–Whitney U test for significant variables. To compare the values of the AIDAI score, the Friedman test was used and, if significant, the Wilcoxon rank sum test. To evaluate the correlation between the serum parameters of inflammation, the Pearson's correlation coefficient was applied.

All data were analyzed using SPSS version 22.0 (SPSS Inc, Chicago, IL, USA) and MedCalc Software (Mariakerke, Belgium).

The study was approved by the Ethics Committee of the University of Palermo, Italy. Informed consent was obtained from all patients who participated in the study.

3. Results

3.1. Clinical Data

During the study period, a total of 995 outpatients with self-reported symptoms on wheat ingestion were examined at the 2 centers. FMF was newly diagnosed in 15 (14 females), equivalent to a prevalence of 1.5% in this population. FMF diagnosis had been previously missed in all these patients.

After excluding 2 patients who were diagnosed with CeD, and 5 patients who tested negative in the DBPC wheat challenge, 8 FMF/NCWS patients were identified. Six of them accepted to enroll in the present study.

These 6 patients tested negative for serum anti-tTG IgA and anti-DGP IgG; four of them tested negative for the HLA DQ2 and DQ8 haplotypes. The 2 HLA DQ2 and DQ8 positive patients underwent duodenal biopsies to exclude a seronegative CeD, and both had normal villi/crypts ratio (>3:1).

All patients were Caucasian, belonged to the Mediterranean population of Southern of Italy, and all carried one of the FMF gene sequence variants, located on chromosome 16.p13.3, encoding the protein pyrin, recorded in Infevers, an online registry of FMF genetic variants. They complained mainly of abdominal pain and diarrhea, and of increased symptoms on wheat ingestion. None of them had been diagnosed with FMF before their referral to us. All had undergone at least one recent gastroscopy and colonoscopy, and CeD, IBD, and IgE-mediated wheat allergy were excluded.

At study start, 4 patients were on colchicine treatment and reported improvement but no resolution of their FMF symptoms; two patients were only on a diet that excluded wheat, as they were asymptomatic on this regimen.

The modified AIDAI score was recorded for 2 weeks before the DBPC challenges, ranging between 4 and 8 points (median 5.5), as none of the patients were completely asymptomatic.

Three patients were initially randomly assigned to wheat and 3 to rice (placebo), to shifted to the other regimen according to the cross-over design. Figure 2A shows the individual AIDAI scores at baseline (on a wheat-free diet) and after the wheat vs. placebo challenges. Under the placebo challenge, the AIDAI score increased slightly (from 5.5 ± 1.5 to 7.0 ± 1.6, mean $\pm$ SD). Under the wheat challenge, however, the score showed a marked increase to 19 ± 6.3 (Figure 2B).

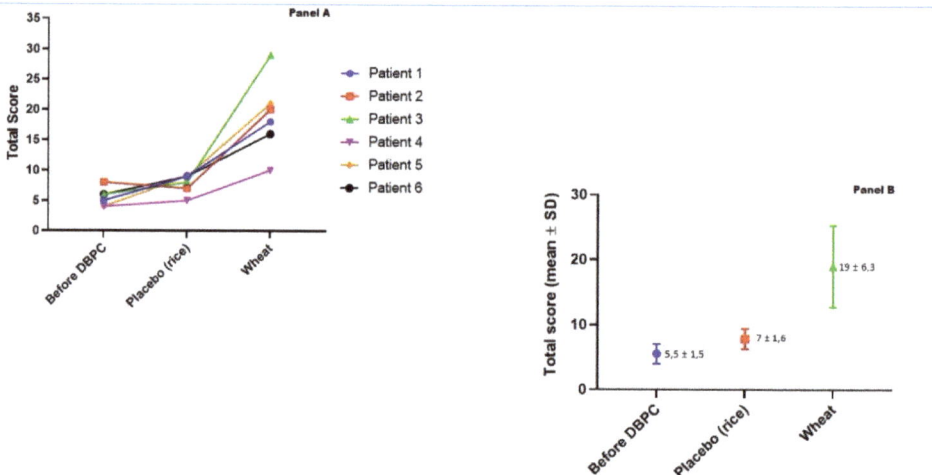

Figure 2. Individual Auto-Inflammatory Diseases Activity Index (AIDAI) scores at baseline and after the placebo and wheat challenges in 6 patients with FMF and NCWS (**A**), and mean values ($\pm$ SD) at baseline and after the placebo and the wheat challenge (**B**).

The difference between the placebo (rice) and the wheat challenge, and between baseline and the wheat challenge were significant (both $p = 0.028$). On the wheat challenge, 3 patients reported fever and 2 did not complete the 2 weeks of the challenge (pts 4 and 5, stopping after 2 and 5 days, respectively), as they developed severe symptoms (fever, diarrhea, vomiting, headache, arthro-myalgias, and skin rash) starting on the first day of wheat consumption. The AIDAI score of these patients was the highest of the whole group, and their scores were included as the last observation put forward (intention-to-treat statistical analysis). The other 4 patients completed the two 14-day challenges, despite increased symptoms during the challenge that finally turned out to be with wheat. In general, symptoms occurred within 1 and 8 days after beginning the wheat challenges (median 3 days). The individual AIDAI score and each sub-score are shown in Supplemental file 3 (Figure S1).

3.2. Serum Markers of Inflammation

Table 1 shows the median and range of sCD14, CRP, and SAA. Mean CRP and SAA serum levels were increased (almost) twofold in FMF patients after the wheat challenge, but this did not reach statistical significance. Compared to HC, FMF patients (before and after the wheat challenge), as well as non-FMF NCWS patients on a wheat-containing diet, showed significantly higher values of sCD14. Considering the whole study population, CRP correlated with SAA ($r = 0.856$; $p < 0.0001$) and with sCD14 ($r = 0.415$; $p = 0.01$).

Table 1. Median and range of soluble CD14 (sCD14), C-reactive protein (CRP), and serum amyloid A (SAA) in the 6 FMF patients at baseline (on a wheat-free diet), at the end of the wheat challenge, and at the end of the placebo (rice) challenge, in 12 patients with symptomatic NCWS and in 8 healthy controls (both on a wheat-containing diet).

	sCD14 (pg/ml)	CRP (mg/L)	SAA (mg/L)
FMF at baseline	11357 (9215–14210)	2.6 (2–9)	6.9 (0.7–26.7)
FMF after wheat challenge	10023 (9112–1436)	5.0 (2–9)	17.3 (2.9–42.7)
FMF after placebo (rice) challenge	11035 (9068–13510)	3.6 (2–5)	12.1 (1.8–27,6)
NCWS patients (on wheat)	11089 (9043–12245)	2.9 (2–7)	6.7 (1.9–38.4)
Healthy controls	8710 (8023–9205)	2.6 (1–4)	4.7 (1.9–34.1)

For sCD14, Kruskall–Wallis test: $p = 0.001$; for other comparisons: Mann–Whitney U test: FMF at baseline vs. HC, $p = 0.002$; FMF after wheat challenge vs. HC, $p = 0.002$; FMF after placebo (rice) challenge vs. HC, $p = 0.002$; NCWS vs. HC, $p = 0.0001$. No other comparisons reached statistical significance.

3.3. Immune Profiling of PBMC by FACS

The percentage of total $CD14^+$ PBMC was similar in FMF patients before the wheat challenge, on wheat-free diet, and in symptomatic NCWS patients on a wheat-containing diet, and significantly higher in both groups compared to the HC (for FMF $p = 0.002$, for NCWS $p = 0.05$). Surprisingly, and in line with the results for serum sCD14 (Table 1), peripheral $CD14^+$ cell counts declined in FMF patients after vs. before wheat challenge ($p = 0.004$); the values after the wheat challenge were also significantly lower than after the placebo challenge ($p = 0.05$) (Figure 3).

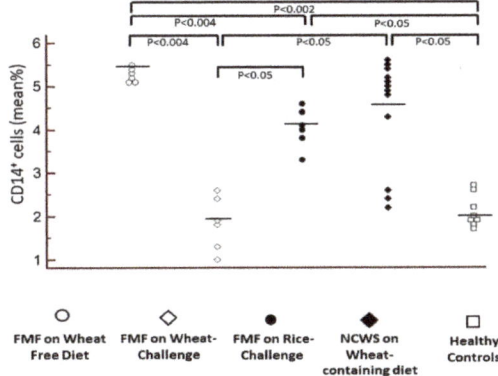

Figure 3. Evaluation of the percentage of $CD14^+$ monocytes in the peripheral blood of the 6 FMF patients with NCWS, before and after the wheat challenge, and after the placebo (rice) challenge, in twelve symptomatic NCWS patients (on a wheat containing diet), and in 8 healthy controls. Symbols indicate the individual values; bars indicate mean values.

However, compared to baseline, the percentage of circulating pro-inflammatory $CD14^+/IL-1\beta^+$ monocytes was significantly increased in FMF patients after the wheat challenge ($p = 0.004$), with values significantly higher than after the placebo challenge ($p = 0.004$) and HC $p = 0.02$). A comparable pattern was seen for CD14$^+$/TNF-α^+ monocytes ($p = 0.004$ vs. baseline, $p = 0.004$ vs. placebo challenge, $p = 0.002$ vs. HC) (Figure 4).

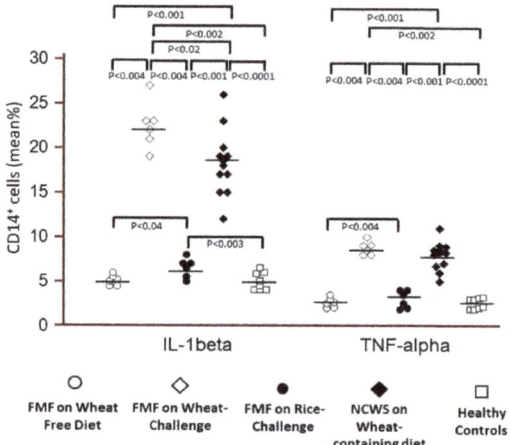

Figure 4. Evaluation of CD14+/IL1-beta+, and CD14+/TNF+ monocytes in the peripheral blood of the 6 FMF patients with NCWS, before and after the wheat challenge and placebo (rice) challenge, in 12 symptomatic NCWS patients (on a wheat containing diet) and in 8 healthy controls.

Interestingly, the 2 patients who did not complete the 2 weeks of the wheat challenge, as they developed severe symptoms and showed the highest AIDAI score of the whole group, were those with the highest percentage of circulating pro-inflammatory CD14$^+$/IL-1β^+ monocytes (Figure 4).

4. Discussion

Although non-celiac gluten sensitivity (NCGS, correctly NCWS) had been described as a distinct clinical condition about 40 years ago [12], it is now identified as a syndrome, characterized by symptoms which can involve the gastrointestinal tract, the nervous system, the skin, the female reproductive tract, and other organs, following the ingestion of gluten/wheat, in subjects who do not suffer from CeD or IgE-mediated wheat allergy [13–15].

However, NCWS is a still ill-defined clinical condition of wheat sensitivity in patients in whom CeD or IgE-mediated wheat allergy have been excluded. Other diseases can overlap with NCWS, in particular some autoimmune and auto-inflammatory conditions that are worsened by wheat ingestion and improve on a wheat ("gluten")-free diet. In this respect, it has been demonstrated that one third of NCWS subjects showed associated autoimmune diseases (such as Hashimoto's thyroiditis) and more than 40% had positive serum anti-nuclear antibodies compared to 2%–6% in the control group including subjects suffering from irritable bowel syndrome [16].

The frequency of FMF among our patients with self-reported NCWS was 1.5%, which is astonishingly high compared to the worldwide prevalence of FMF, estimated at 1:100,000–150,000, with the highest prevalence in non-Ashkenazi Jews or Armenians, estimated at 1:250–500, groups, that were not represented in our cohort [17]. Therefore, in populations with a higher, but also with a lower prevalence of FMF, we need to consider the diagnosis of NCWS combined with FMF, an otherwise rare disease that is often overlooked in clinical practice.

It must be underlined that FMF diagnosis had been missed previously in all the patients included in our study; this could be due to the rarity of this disease and the consequent low awareness by physicians. Therefore, both internists and gastroenterologists should consider this diagnosis also in patients with self-reported NCWS and abdominal and general inflammatory symptoms.

During the DBPC challenge of the present study, all the enrolled patients relapsed on the wheat challenge, to show an AIDAI score significantly higher with the wheat challenge than at baseline or with the placebo challenge. Symptom relapse was so severe that 2 patients interrupted the challenge on the 3rd and 6th day, respectively, and 3 patients developed fever (>38°C). None of them reacted to the placebo (rice) challenge.

We found that serum levels of sCD14 were significantly higher in FMF-NCWS patients than in HC, with levels comparable to patients with NCWS alone. In FMF-NCWS patients, sCD14 levels did not increase after the wheat challenge compared to baseline, suggesting a stable pro-inflammatory predisposition and, perhaps, a tissue recruitment towards serosal tissues after wheat exposure. Notably, the number of circulating $CD14^+/IL-1\beta^+$ and $CD14^+/TNF-\alpha^+$ monocytes increased significantly in the FMF patients 12 h after the wheat challenge, compared with baseline and with the placebo (rice) challenge. In view of decreased total CD14+ cells, this suggests a dramatic increase in the proportion of pro-inflammatory vs. non-activated monocytes in the circulation, considered a hallmark of (auto-)inflammation. Their values after the wheat challenge were also significantly higher than in HC. Notably, increased IL-1β and TNF-α^+ production by monocytes are considered hallmarks of innate immune activation and consequent inflammation in FMF [18], and possibly also in the pathogenesis of NCWS [19].

Our findings are in accord with prior reports that stressed the impact of environmental factors on the course of FMF [20], although no defined triggers had been identified so far.

The findings of the present study are well in agreement also with our prior experimental data that showed that a specific non-gluten protein component of wheat, the family of ATIs, activate innate immunity in the gut [21,22]. ATIs engage the toll-like receptor 4 (TLR4)-MD2-CD14 complex, leading to an upregulation of monocyte, macrophage, and especially dendritic cell maturation markers and an increased release of pro-inflammatory cytokines and chemokines by these myeloid cells [23]. Furthermore, it has been demonstrated that a wheat-, and therefore, ATI-containing diet worsened IBD, as well as nutritional and inhalative allergies [10,21,24]. Moreover, our unpublished results in mouse models of autoimmune diseases, such as multiple sclerosis or systemic lupus erythematosus, indicate that nutritional ATIs worsen ongoing chronic inflammatory diseases in general [25]. In the mentioned studies, IL-1β and TNF-α^+ were central mediators of myeloid cell activation that was triggered in the intestine (and the periphery) by wheat ATIs. We therefore suggest that ATIs may be the primary "culprits" in wheat that activate innate immunity and exacerbates FMF [21–23].

Our study has some limitations. First, it is a pilot study, including a low number of patients. However, FMF is a rare disorder and we are planning further studies, involving a much higher number of FMF patients, and considering a broad range of biological parameters. The completion of the planned studies, however, will take several years and we consider it unethical to withhold publication of the present study that shows a spectrum of significant results, despite the low number of patients.

Second, we observed the association between wheat consumption and FMF in 2 tertiary centers that are dedicated to wheat and nutrition-related diseases. Consequently, the high frequency of FMF patients with self-reported NCWS, and the association of FMF with NCWS may have been overestimated. Thus, we were not able to evaluate the overall therapeutic contribution of a wheat-free diet in FMF.

Third, other wheat-related components and mechanisms may add to the worsening of intestinal symptoms in our FMF patients exposed to wheat. Such a mechanistically different inflammatory condition that causes abdominal symptoms could be "atypical" food allergies, prominently to wheat, suggested by recent histological [9] and confocal endomicroscopy studies [26,27].

Fourth, the intestinal microbiota, as affected by wheat compared to a wheat-free diet, may be an important environmental factor affecting the severity of FMF [28]. But here again, we could demonstrate the wheat ATI can directly promote intestinal pro-inflammatory dysbiosis [29].

Finally, we focused only on the role of IL-1β and TNF-α production by PBMC, but likely, there is also a role for IL-6, IL-17, IL-22, and other cytokines, as it has been suggested in other studies on FMF patients [30].

5. Conclusions

Our pilot study provides the first evidence that self-reported symptoms due to wheat ingestion can reveal a FMF diagnosis previously missed, and that wheat ingestion can lead to immune activation and exacerbation of FMF. The subgroup of FMF patients who can benefit from a wheat-free diet needs to be well-defined in future studies. In this subgroup of patients, it is possible that a wheat-free diet could become a cornerstone for treatment and prevention of FMF. In general, however, regardless of the patients' subjective feelings about the severity of their fever and pain attacks, it is advisable to continue colchicine therapy at adequate doses to prevent the one life-threatening complications of FMF, such as amyloidosis.

Supplementary Materials: The following are available online at http://www.mdpi.com/2072-6643/12/4/1127/s1, Table S1: Demographic and clinical characteristics of the 6 FMF patients included; file 2: AIDAI score form for the patients; file 3: Representative FACS plots showing the gating strategy used to analyze expression of the pro-inflammatory cytokines IL-1b and TNF-a by CD14+ monocytes obtained from the peripheral of a FMF patient on the wheat-free diet. Blue: isotype control mAb. Pink: cytokine-specific mAb; Figure S1: Individual ADAI scores of the FMF-NCWS patients at baseline, and after wheat or rice (placebo) challenge.

Author Contributions: A.C., P.M., D.S., and D.D.L. had full access to all of the data in the study and take responsibility for the integrity of the data and the accuracy of the data analysis. Conceptualization: A.C. Data curation: A.C., P.M., F.L.B., M.S. Investigation: Endoscopy study: G.G. Investigation: Cell and Cytokine analyses: F.D., D.D.L., F.F., M.L.P. Investigation: Markers of inflammation: E.M., D.S. Investigation: Genetic studies: A.P. Software: M.S. Format Analysis: A.C., D.D.L., D.S. Writing-original draft: A.C., D.D.L., D.S. Writing-Review & Editing: A.C., D.S. All authors have read and agreed to the published version of the manuscript.

Funding: AC is supported by the Italian Health Ministry, Grant PE-2016-02363692 and by the Italian Foundation for Celiac Disease (AIC) Grant for Project 013 2014. DS is supported by research grants from the German Research Foundation DFG Schu 646/17-1 (ATI), DFG Pic/Sch SPP 1656 (Intestinal microbiota), DFG Schu 646/20-1 (Allergy), Collaborative Research Center 128 A08 (Multiple sclerosis), and from the Leibniz Foundation (Wheatscan, SAW-2016-DFA-2). The study sponsors, listed in the Acknowledgement, had no role in study design, in the collection, analysis and interpretation of the data, in writing the manuscript and in the decision to submit the paper for publication.

Acknowledgments: We wish to thank all the patients who agreed to participate in the study.

Conflicts of Interest: The authors declare that there are no conflicts of interests regarding publication of this paper.

Registration: The study was registered at Clinicaltrials.gov (registration number NCT03563300), accessible at: https://www.clinicaltrials.gov/ct2/show/NCT03563300?term=wheat&cond=Familial+Mediterranean+Fever&draw=2&rank=1).

Abbreviations

AIDAI	Auto-Inflammatory Disease Activity Index
CeD	Celiac Disease
CRP	C-Reactive Protein
DBPC	Double-Blind Placebo-Controlled
FABP2	Fatty Acid-Binding Protein 2
FMF	Familial Mediterranean Fever
LBP	Lipopolysaccharide-Binding Protein
NCWS	Non-Celiac Wheat Sensitivity
PBMC	Peripheral Blood Monocytes Cells
SAA	Serum Amyloid A
sCD14	soluble CD14
SD	Standard Deviation

References

1. Sapone, A.; Bai, J.C.; Ciacci, C.; Dolinsek, J.; Green, P.H.; Hadjivassiliou, M.; Kaukinen, K.; Rostami, K.; Sanders, D.S.; Schumann, M. Spectrum of gluten-related disorders: Consensus on new nomenclature and classification. *BMC. Med.* **2012**. [CrossRef]
2. Catassi, C.; Alaedini, A.; Bojarski, C.; Bonaz, B.; Bouma, G.; Carroccio, A.; Castillejo, G.; De Magistris, L.; Dieterich, W.; Di Liberto, D. The Overlapping Area of Non-Celiac Gluten Sensitivity (NCGS) and Wheat-Sensitive Irritable Bowel Syndrome (IBS): An Update. *Nutrients* **2017**, *9*. [CrossRef] [PubMed]
3. Catassi, C.; Elli, L.; Bonaz, B.; Bouma, G.; Carroccio, A.; Castillejo, G.; Cellier, C.; Cristofori, F.; De Magistris, L.; Dolinsek, J. Diagnosis of Non-Celiac Gluten Sensitivity (NCGS): The Salerno Experts' Criteria. *Nutrients* **2015**, *7*, 4966–4977. [CrossRef] [PubMed]
4. Uhde, M.; Ajamian, M.; Caio, G.; De Giorgio, R.; Indart, A.; Green, P.H.; Verna, E.C.; Volta, U.; Alaedini, A. Intestinal cell damage and systemic immune activation in individuals reporting sensitivity to wheat in the absence of coeliac disease. *Gut* **2016**, *65*, 1930–1937. [CrossRef] [PubMed]
5. Demir, A.; Akyüz, F.; Göktürk, S.; Evirgen, S.; Akyüz, U.; Örmeci, A.; Soyer, O.; Karaca, C.; Demir, K.; Gundogdu, G. Small bowel mucosal damage in familial Mediterranean fever: Results of capsule endoscopy screening. *Scand. J. Gastroenterol.* **2014**, *49*, 1414–1418. [CrossRef]
6. Berkun, Y.; Eisenstein, E.M. Diagnostic criteria of familial Mediterranean fever. *Autoimmun. Rev.* **2014**, *13*, 388–390. [CrossRef]
7. Zemer, D.; Pras, M.; Sohar, E.; Gafni, J. Letter: Colchicine in familial Mediterranean fever. *N. Engl. J. Med.* **1976**, *294*, 170–171. [CrossRef]
8. Livneh, A.; Langevitz, P.; Zemer, D.; Zaks, N.; Kees, S.; Lidar, T.; Migdal, A.; Padeh, S.; Pras, M. Criteria for the diagnosis of familial Mediterranean fever. *Arthritis Rheum.* **1997**, *40*, 1879–1885. [CrossRef]
9. Carroccio, A.; Giannone, G.; Mansueto, P.; Soresi, M.; La Blasca, F.; Fayer, F.; Iacobucci, R.; Porcasi, R.; Catalano, T.; Geraci, G. Duodenal and Rectal Mucosa Inflammation in Patients With Non-celiac Wheat Sensitivity. *Clin. Gastroenterol. Hepatol.* **2019**, *17*, 682–690. [CrossRef]
10. Zevallos, V.F.; Raker, V.K.; Maxeiner, J.; Scholtes, P.; Steinbrink, K.; Schuppan, D. Dietary wheat amylase trypsin inhibitors exacerbate murine allergic airway inflammation. *Eur. J. Nutr.* **2019**, *58*, 1507–1514. [CrossRef]
11. Piram, M.; Koné-Paut, I.; Lachmann, H.J.; Frenkel, J.; Ozen, S.; Kuemmerle-Deschner, J.; Stojanov, S.; Simon, A.; Finetti, M.; Sormani, M.P. Validation of the auto-inflammatory diseases activity index (AIDAI) for hereditary recurrent fever syndromes. *Ann. Rheum. Dis.* **2014**, *73*, 2168–2173. [CrossRef] [PubMed]
12. Ellis, A.; Linaker, B.D. Non Celiac Gluten Sensitivity. *Lancet.* **1978**, *1*, 1386–1389. [CrossRef]
13. Mansueto, P.; Seidita, A.; D'Alcamo, A.; Carroccio, A. Non-celiac gluten sensitivity: Literature review. *J. Am. Coll. Nutr.* **2014**, *33*, 39–54. [CrossRef] [PubMed]
14. Elli, L.; Villalta, D.; Roncoroni, L.; Barisani, D.; Ferrero, S.; Pellegrini, N.; Bardella, M.T.; Valiante, F.; Tomba, C.; Carroccio, A. Nomenclature and diagnosis of gluten-related disorders: A position statement by the Italian Association of Hospital Gastroenterologists and Endoscopists (AIGO). *Dig. Liver Dis.* **2017**, *49*, 138–146. [CrossRef] [PubMed]
15. Volta, U.; Caio, G.; Karunaratne, T.B.; Alaedini, A.; De Giorgio, R. Non-coeliac gluten/wheat sensitivity: Advances in knowledge and relevant questions. *Expert. Rev. Gastroenterol. Hepatol.* **2017**, *11*, 9–18. [CrossRef]
16. Carroccio, A.; D'Alcamo, A.; Cavataio, F.; Soresi, M.; Seidita, A.; Sciumè, C.; Geraci, G.; Iacono, G.; Mansueto, P. High Proportions of People With Nonceliac Wheat Sensitivity Have Autoimmune Disease or Antinuclear Antibodies. *Gastroenterology* **2015**, *149*, 596–603. [CrossRef]
17. Portincasa, P.; Scaccianoce, G.; Palasciano, G. Familial mediterranean fever: A fascinating model of inherited autoinflammatory disorder. *Eur. J. Clin. Investig.* **2013**, *43*, 1314–1327. [CrossRef]
18. Stojanov, S.; Kastner, D.L. Familial autoinflammatory diseases: Genetics, pathogenesis and treatment. *Curr. Opin. Rheumatol.* **2005**, *17*, 586–599. [CrossRef]
19. Sapone, A.; Lammers, K.M.; Casolaro, V.; Cammarota, M.; Giuliano, M.T.; De Rosa, M.; Stefanile, R.; Mazzarella, G.; Tolone, C.; Russo, M.I. Divergence of gut permeability and mucosal immune gene expression in two gluten-associated conditions: Celiac disease and gluten sensitivity. *BMC. Med.* **2011**, *9*, 23. [CrossRef]
20. Ozen, S.; Batu, E.D. The myths we believed in familial Mediterranean fever: What have we learned in the past years? *Semin. Immunopathol.* **2015**, *37*, 363–369. [CrossRef]

21. Zevallos, V.F.; Raker, V.; Tenzer, S.; Jimenez-Calvente, C.; Ashfaq-Khan, M.; Rüssel, N.; Pickert, G.; Schild, H.; Steinbrink, K.; Schuppan, D. Nutritional wheat amylase-trypsin inhibitors promote intestinal inflammation via activation of myeloid cells. *Gastroenterology* **2017**, *152*, 1100–1113. [CrossRef]
22. Caminero, A.; McCarville, J.L.; Zevallos, V.F.; Pigrau, M.; Yu, X.B.; Jury, J.; Galipeau, H.J.; Clarizio, A.V.; Casqueiro, J.; Murray, J.A. Lactobacilli degrade wheat amylase trypsin inhibitors to reduce intestinal dysfunction induced by immunogenic wheat proteins. *Gastroenterology* **2019**, *156*, 2266–2280. [CrossRef]
23. Junker, Y.; Zeissig, S.; Kim, S.J.; Barisani, D.; Wieser, H.; Leffler, D.A.; Zevallos, V.; Libermann, T.A.; Dillon, S.; Freitag, T.L. Wheat amylase trypsin inhibitors drive intestinal inflammation via activation of toll-like receptor 4. *J. Exp. Med.* **2012**, *209*, 2395–2408. [CrossRef] [PubMed]
24. Bellinghausen, I.; Weigmann, B.; Zevallos, V.; Maxeiner, J.; Reißig, S.; Waisman, A.; Schuppan, D.; Saloga, J. Wheat amylase-trypsin inhibitors exacerbate intestinal and airway allergic immune responses in humanized mice. *J. Allergy Clin. Immunol.* **2019**, *143*, 201–212. [CrossRef]
25. Schuppan, D.; Pickert, G.; Ashfaq-Khan, M.; Zevallos, V. Non-celiac wheat sensitivity: Differential diagnosis, triggers and implications. Best. *Pract. Res. Clin. Gastroenterol.* **2015**, *29*, 469–476. [CrossRef] [PubMed]
26. Fritscher-Ravens, A.; Pflaum, T.; Mösinger, M.; Ruchay, Z.; Röcken, C.; Milla, P.J.; Das, M.; Bottner, M.; Wedel, T.; Schuppan, D. Many Patients With Irritable Bowel Syndrome Have Atypical Food Allergies Not Associated With Immunoglobulin E. *Gastroenterology* **2019**, *157*, 109–118. [CrossRef] [PubMed]
27. Fritscher-Ravens, A.; Schuppan, D.; Ellrichmann, M.; Schoch, S.; Röcken, C.; Brasch, J.; Bethge, J.; Bottner, M.; Klose, J.; Milla, P.J. Confocal endomicroscopy shows food-associated changes in the intestinal mucosa of patients with irritable bowel syndrome. *Gastroenterology* **2014**, *147*, 1012–1020. [CrossRef] [PubMed]
28. Luken, J.R.; Gurung, P.; Vogel, P.; Johnson, G.R.; Carter, R.A.; McGoldrick, D.J.; Bandi, S.R.; Calabrese, C.R.; Walle, L.V.; Lamkanfi, M. Dietary modulation of the microbiome affects autoinflammatory disease. *Nature* **2014**, *516*, 246–249. [CrossRef]
29. Pickert, G.; Wirtz, S.; Matzner, J.; AshfaqKhan, M.; Heck, R.; Rosigkeit, S.; Thies, D.; Surabattula, R.; Ehmann, D.; Wehkamp, J.; et al. Wheat consumption aggravates experimental colitis by amylase trypsin inhibitor (ATI)-mediated dysbiosis. *Gastroenterology* **2020**, in press. [CrossRef]
30. Ibrahim, J.N.; Jounblat, R.; Delwail, A.; Abou-Ghoch, J.; Salem, N.; Chouery, E.; Megarbane, A.; Medlej-Hashim, M.; Lecron, J.C. Ex vivo PBMC cytokine profile in familial Mediterranean fever patients: Involvement of IL-1β, IL-1α and Th17-associated cytokines and decrease of Th1 and Th2 cytokines. *Cytokine* **2014**, *69*, 248–254. [CrossRef]

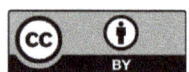

© 2020 by the authors. Licensee MDPI, Basel, Switzerland. This article is an open access article distributed under the terms and conditions of the Creative Commons Attribution (CC BY) license (http://creativecommons.org/licenses/by/4.0/).

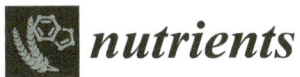

Communication

Irritable Bowel Syndrome and Gluten-Related Disorders

Paolo Usai-Satta [1,*], Gabrio Bassotti [2], Massimo Bellini [3], Francesco Oppia [1], Mariantonia Lai [4] and Francesco Cabras [1]

1. Gastroenterology Unit, Brotzu Hospital, 09121 Cagliari, Italy; f.oppia@tiscali.it (F.O.); francescocabras@aob.it (F.C.)
2. Gastroenterology & Hepatology Section, Department of Medicine, University of Perugia, 06156 Perugia, Italy; gabassot@tin.it
3. Gastrointestinal Unit, Department of Translational Research and New Technologies in Medicine and Surgery, University of Pisa, 56010 Pisa, Italy; mbellini58@gmail.com
4. Gastroenterology Unit, University of Cagliari, 09042 Monserrato, Italy; marlai@aoucagliari.it
* Correspondence: paolousai@aob.it; Tel.: +39-070-539-395

Received: 22 March 2020; Accepted: 13 April 2020; Published: 17 April 2020

Abstract: Background: Irritable bowel syndrome (IBS) is frequently associated with celiac disease (CD) and nonceliac gluten/wheat sensitivity (NCGS/NCWS), but epidemiological and pathophysiological aspects are still unclear. Furthermore, a gluten-free diet (GFD) can positively influence IBS symptoms. **Methods**: A comprehensive online search for IBS related to CD, NCGS and GFD was made using the Pubmed, Medline and Cochrane databases. **Results**: Although a systematic screening for CD in IBS is not recommended, CD prevalence can be increased in diarrhea-predominant IBS patients. On the other hand, IBS symptoms can be persistent in treated CD patients, and their prevalence tends to decrease on a GFD. IBS symptoms may overlap and be similar to those associated to nonceliac gluten and/or wheat sensitivity. Increased gut permeability could explain the gluten/wheat effects in IBS patients. Finally, a GFD could improve symptoms in a subgroup of IBS patients. **Conclusions**: The possible interplay between IBS and gluten-related disorders represents a scientifically and clinically challenging issue. Further studies are needed to confirm these data and better clarify the involved pathophysiological mechanisms.

Keywords: irritable bowel syndrome; celiac disease; nonceliac gluten/wheat sensitivity; gluten-free diet

1. Introduction

Irritable bowel syndrome (IBS) is the most frequently diagnosed functional gastrointestinal disorder, causing abdominal pain, bloating, diarrhea and constipation [1]. This condition affects 10–15% of the general population and is associated with a decreased quality of life (QoL). IBS is classified into three main subtypes according to the predominant bowel habit: constipation-predominant (IBS-C), diarrhea-predominant (IBS-D) and mixed bowel habits (IBS-M) [2–6]. Since there are no available biological markers that clearly identify such patients, the diagnosis of IBS is usually made based on the symptoms according to the Rome IV criteria [7]. These criteria suggest performing limited laboratory studies, including serological tests for celiac disease (CD) in patients with IBS-D and IBS-M. The initial treatment is directed towards lifestyle and, eventually, dietary modification. Subsequently, an appropriate pharmacotherapy can be proposed [8].

Although a mutual relationship between CD and IBS has been hypothesized, the available evidence is controversial [9,10]. In addition, the symptom complex of IBS-D may overlap and resemble that associated with nonceliac gluten/wheat sensitivity (NCGS/NCWS) [11]. Finally, a gluten-free diet (GFD) has been proposed in a subgroup of patients with IBS as a possible therapeutic option [12]. This review aimed to evaluate and clarify the relationship between IBS and gluten-related disorders, including the impact of a GFD in IBS patients.

2. Materials and Methods

We performed a comprehensive online search of Medline, Cochrane and the Science Citation Index using the keywords "irritable bowel syndrome", "celiac disease", "non celiac gluten sensitivity" and "gluten free diet" in various combinations with the Boolean operators *and*, *or*, and *not*, selecting articles published in English between January 2000 and December 2019.

3. IBS and CD

CD is a chronic, gluten-related disorder characterized by small intestinal mucosal inflammation and malabsorption in genetically predisposed individuals. The prevalence of CD in the worldwide general population is reported to be about 1% [13,14]. The clinical picture of CD often overlaps with that of IBS, and several studies suggest that IBS patients are at increased risk of CD [9,15]. In contrast to IBS, symptoms may resolve if the disease is recognized and a strict GFD is respected. However, sufficient data are not available to demonstrate a higher prevalence of CD in patients with IBS-D compared with those with IBS-C or IBS-M. International guidelines yield conflicting recommendations about systematic screening for CD in IBS individuals [16–18]. From 2002 to 2007, the American Gastroenterological Association and the British Society of Gastroenterology suggested limited serological tests, whereas the American College of Gastroenterology did not recommend any laboratory investigations. A meta-analysis by Ford et al. [15] included 14 studies, comprising 4204 individuals. The prevalence of histology-proven CD in IBS patients was more than four-fold that in controls without IBS. A more recent meta-analysis [9] included 36 eligible studies, comprising 9275 subjects meeting the criteria for IBS. Pooled odds ratios (ORs) for positive antiendomysial antibodies (EMA) and/or tissue transglutaminase antibodies (tTG), and histology-proven CD in IBS subjects versus controls were 2.75 (95% CI 1.35–5.61), and 4.48 (95% CI 2.33–8.60). The prevalence of biopsy-positive CD was significantly higher across all subtypes of IBS. Also, the Rome IV foundation suggested that serologic tests for CD should be performed in patients with IBS-D and IBS-M who fail empiric therapy [7]. According to recent Canadian guidelines [6], testing for CD could be suggested in IBS-D rather than in IBS-C patients, although the studies concerning the role of celiac testing in IBS were of low-quality. On the other hand, studies from the United States [9,19], including a recent AGA technical review [5], did not identify an increase in the prevalence or in the ORs of CD in patients with IBS. In any case, universal screening for CD in every IBS patient is presently not recommended.

4. CD and IBS

Clinical practice suggests that many patients with CD have persistent digestive symptoms despite long-term GFD. Such (a) persistence of symptoms notwithstanding, strict dietary restrictions, is frustrating and may even lead to poor dietary adherence. More solid data on these clinical findings would be useful to improve the management and follow-up of celiac patients.

Several studies have suggested that the prevalence of IBS symptoms among patients with CD on GFD may be higher than in the general population [20,21], but no conclusive data are available about the actual prevalence of functional gastrointestinal disorders in patients with CD. In addition, the association with autoimmune diseases, microscopic colitis, or small intestinal bacterial overgrowth may be a further diagnostic confounding factor [13]. Barratt et al. [22] showed that IBS is more prevalent in CD on GFD in comparison with age-matched and sex-matched controls. The prevalence of IBS in CD was 22%. IBS additional symptoms were associated with reduced QoL and an increased likelihood of anxiety and depression. In 2013, a meta-analysis [10] showed a pooled prevalence of IBS symptoms of 38% (95% CI, 27.0–50.0%) in all patients with CD. Furthermore, celiac patients displayed a pooled OR for IBS symptoms that was higher than controls (5.60; 95% CI, 3.23–9.70). Improved adherence to a GFD might be associated with a reduction in symptoms. A more recent study [23] evaluated the prevalence and severity of IBS symptoms related to GFD in a group of CD patients. Based on a variable duration of GFD, patients were classified into short-term GFD (one to two years) and long-term GFD (greater than three years) groups and compared with a group of healthy controls. Although there were no differences in symptoms between the short- and long-term GFD groups, both had a worse symptom score than controls ($p = 0.03$ and $p = 0.05$, respectively). In another recent study [24] adult CD patients were studied at diagnosis, six months, and one year after GFD using Rome III criteria for IBS. At diagnosis and after one year of GFD, 52% and 22% of patients fulfilled the criteria for IBS, respectively. Therefore, IBS was persistent in treated CD patients, but its prevalence significantly decreased on a GFD.

5. IBS, Gluten, Wheat, and NCGS/NCWS

The presence of intestinal and extraintestinal symptoms related to gluten-containing food without the diagnostic findings of CD or wheat allergy has recently been named nonceliac gluten sensitivity (NCGS) [25]. Unlike CD, NCGS has no available specific diagnostic markers [26]. The complex of digestive symptoms associated with NCGS, such as diarrhea, bloating, or abdominal pain, may overlap and be similar to those caused by IBS-D [11]. The main difference between NCGS and IBS is usually based on the fact that patients with NCGS self-report symptoms when consuming gluten. Conversely, IBS patients generally do not report gluten ingestion as a specific stimulus for their symptoms [27]. However, food plays an important provocative role in IBS symptoms, and up to 80% of IBS patients complain of postprandial discomfort. Furthermore, many patients report presumed food intolerances [28,29]. According to recent evidence, the spectrum of symptoms that occur in NCGS patients may be due not only to gluten proteins, but also to other wheat-related components. Therefore, the term nonceliac wheat sensitivity (NCWS) has been coined [30,31]. Wheat contains a number of nongluten compounds that could produce digestive symptoms. Some of these compounds could be related to FODMAPS (fermentable oligo-, di-, and monosaccharides and polyols), specifically fructans [32]. The mechanism by which wheat or specific wheat components such as gluten cause IBS-type symptoms remains debatable [33]. In a study using confocal endomicroscopy, wheat administered endoscopically into the duodenal mucosa was able to affect the small intestinal mucosa integrity [34]. In a more recent study, intestinal permeability was significantly increased after gluten challenge in a group of gluten-sensitive, nonceliac IBS-D patients [35].

It can thus be hypothesized that an incomplete degradation of gluten and other wheat proteins allows undigested peptides to cross a more permeable mucosal barrier and provoke symptoms. This pathophysiological mechanism could be present at least in a subset of patients with IBS [36,37]. On the other hand, the incomplete knowledge of the pathogenesis and pathophysiology of IBS and NCGS/NCWS does not clarify whether these entities are separate, related, or overlap. Table 1 summarizes the most significant evidence on IBS related to gluten, wheat, and NCGS/NCWS.

Table 1. Summary of the most significant studies on IBS related to gluten/wheat and NCGS/NCWS.

Authors (Ref)	Study Design	Study Method	Participants	Results
Potter [31]	Population-based study	Multivariate analysis	3115	NCWS was associated with IBS (OR: 3.55)
Fritscher–Ravens [34]	Prospective controlled study	Confocal endomicroscopy before and after wheat administration	36 IBS	IEL and intervillous spaces increased after wheat endoscopic challenge
Wu [35]	Double-blinded gluten challenge	Immuno-histochemistry by endoscopic biopsies	27 IBS-D	Increased gut permeability after gluten challenge
Elli [36]	Double-blinded trial	GFD and gluten challenge	134 with functional disorders (77 IBS)	14% of patients meet NCGS criteria
Carroccio [37]	Double-blinded trial	Wheat-free diet and wheat challenge	920 IBS	70 IBS with NCWS

Notes: IBS-D: irritable bowel syndrome with diarrhea, GFD: gluten-free diet, NCGS: nonceliac gluten sensitivity, NCWS: nonceliac wheat sensitivity, OR: odds ratio.

6. IBS and Gluten/Wheat-Free Diet

Based on the above evidence, a gluten- (and also wheat-) free diet appears to represent a potential and appealing dietary intervention for a subset of patients with IBS [38]. There are several double-blind, placebo-controlled and randomized clinical trials evaluating the effect of GFD on IBS. Table 2 summarizes the most significant studies on this topic.

Table 2. Summary of the most significant studies on gluten and wheat-free diet in IBS.

Authors (Ref)	Study Design	Study Duration	Participants	Diet Methods	Results
Vasquez Roque [39]	RCT	6 months	45 IBS-D	GFD and gluten challenge	More bowel movements on gluten challenge
Aziz [40]	Prospective study	6 weeks	41 IBS-D	GFD	Symptoms improved on GFD
Zanwar [41]	DBP trial	4 weeks	60 IBS-D	GFD and gluten challenge	Symptoms worsened on gluten challenge
Elli [36]	DBP trial	3-week GFD, followed by 1-week gluten challenge	77 IBS	GFD and gluten challenge	Symptoms improved in 71% of IBS (34% relapsed on gluten challenge)
Roncoroni [42]	RCT	21 days	50 celiac patients with IBS symptoms	GFD-LFD	Better symptom impact in GFD-LFD than GFD alone
Biesiekierski [30]	DBP trial	2-week LFD, followed by 1 week low, high gluten or placebo	37 IBS-NCGS	High and low gluten challenge	No gluten effect on IBS symptoms; wheat sensitivity hypothesized
Carroccio [37]	DBP trial	5 weeks	276 IBS and wheat sensitivity	Wheat-free diet and wheat challenge	Asymptomatic on wheat-free diet and symptoms increased on wheat challenge
Dionne [12]	Meta-analysis	Variable	111 GFD 397 LFD	GFD and LFD	Low evidence on GFD in IBS

Notes: DBP: double-blinded placebo-controlled, RCT: randomized clinical trial, IBS-D: irritable bowel syndrome with diarrhea, GFD: gluten-free diet, LFD: low FODMAP diet; NCGS: nonceliac gluten sensitivity.

A total of 60 IBS patients completed a double-blind randomized placebo-controlled study [41], in which the recruited subjects underwent GFD for four weeks, followed by a rechallenge of gluten-free bread or cereal-containing bread. This study showed that the gluten challenge group had higher symptom scores. A randomized clinical trial [39] was instead carried out in 45 patients with IBS-D, whose participants underwent either a four-week trial of a GFD or a gluten-containing diet. The authors demonstrated that daily bowel movements increased in patients assuming a gluten-containing diet. Another study [40] performed in 41 patients also showed a significant reduction in IBS-Symptom Severity Score ($p < 0.001$) in IBS-D patients after a six-week GFD. An Italian multicenter study [36] achieved a symptomatic improvement in 55 out 77 IBS patients (71.4%) after a three-week GFD, followed by a double-blind gluten challenge versus placebo, in which 18 out 53 responder patients with IBS (34%) had symptom relapse. Recently [42], a combination of low FODMAP diet and GFD (LFD-GFD) had positive effects in patients with CD and coexisting functional digestive symptoms.

The authors observed a significant reduction in the VAS (visual analog scale) for abdominal pain in the LFD-GFD group versus the normal GFD group ($p < 0.01$).

Concerning gluten as part of the wheat structure, wheat sensitivity has also been hypothesized in IBS patients. A large study [37] including 920 IBS patients with a self-reduced wheat diet performed an elimination diet for four weeks, followed by a double-blind, placebo-controlled challenge. The results showed that 30% of patients had NCWS, and were asymptomatic on an elimination diet. On the other hand, a double-blind placebo-controlled crossover trial [30] showed that participants with self-reported NCGS (and IBS symptoms) following a GFD reported further improved symptoms by LFD, and no specific effects of gluten were found. In a recent meta-analysis [12] including nine studies, GFD was associated with reduced global IBS symptoms compared with a control diet (RR = 0.42; 95% CI 0.11 to 1.55; I2 = 88%), although this was not statistically significant. The authors concluded that the available scientific evidence was not sufficient to recommend a GFD to improve IBS symptoms. According to the most recent evidence, recent Canadian guidelines [6] on the IBS management recommend against GFD in the treatment of IBS.

7. Conclusions

The mutual interplay between IBS and gluten-related disorders represents a topic of increasing interest. Although the prevalence of CD may be increased in IBS-D patients, universal screening for CD is not presently recommended in these patients. However, some evidence shows that in patients with CD on GFD, the persistence of digestive symptoms can be related to IBS. Moreover, the clinical picture of IBS can overlap with NCGS and NCWS, and an increased bowel permeability could explain the mechanism by which gluten and/or wheat can provoke symptoms in IBS subjects. Finally, GFD could decrease the impact of symptoms in a subset of IBS patients. Further studies are needed to assess the role of gluten-related disorders in IBS and vice versa.

Author Contributions: All authors provided input on the content of the manuscript. All authors have read and agreed to the published version of the manuscript.

Funding: This review received no external funding.

Conflicts of Interest: The authors declare no conflict of interest.

References

1. Ford, A.C.; Lacy, B.E.; Talley, N.J. Irritable Bowel Syndrome. *N. Engl. J. Med.* **2017**, *376*, 2566–2578. [CrossRef]
2. Hungin, A.P.S.; Whorwell, P.; Tack, J.; Mearin, F. The prevalence, patterns and impact of irritable bowel syndrome: An international survey of 40 000 subjects. *Aliment. Pharmacol. Ther.* **2003**, *17*, 643–650. [CrossRef]
3. Bellini, M.; Gambaccini, D.; Stasi, C.; Urbano, M.T.; Marchi, S.; Usai-Satta, P. Irritable bowel syndrome: A disease still searching for pathogenesis, diagnosis and therapy. *World J. Gastroenterol.* **2014**, *20*, 8807–8820. [PubMed]
4. Ford, A.C.; Forman, D.; Bailey, A.G.; Axon, A.T.R.; Moayyedi, P. Irritable bowel syndrome: A 10-year natural history of symptoms, and factors that influence consultation behavior. *Am. J. Gastroenterol.* **2008**, *103*, 1229–1239. [CrossRef] [PubMed]
5. Carrasco-Labra, A.; Lytvyn, L.; Falck-Ytter, Y.; Surawicz, C.M.; Chey, W.D. AGA Technical Review on the Evaluation of Functional Diarrhea and Diarrhea-Predominant Irritable Bowel Syndrome in Adults (IBS-D). *Gastroenterology* **2019**, *157*, 859–880. [CrossRef] [PubMed]
6. Moayyedi, P.; Andrews, C.N.; MacQueen, G.; Korownyk, C.; Marsiglio, M.; Graff, L.; Kvern, B.; Lazarescu, A.; Liu, L.; Paterson, W.G.; et al. Canadian Association of Gastroenterology Clinical Practice Guideline for the Management of Irritable Bowel Syndrome (IBS). *J. Can. Assoc. Gastroenterol.* **2019**, *2*, 6–29. [CrossRef]
7. Lacy, B.E.; Mearin, F.; Chang, L.; Chey, W.D.; Lembo, A.J.; Simrén, M.; Spiller, R.C. Bowel Disorders. *Gastroenterology* **2016**, *150*, 1393–1407.e5. [CrossRef]
8. Soncini, M.; Stasi, C.; Usai-Satta, P.; Milazzo, G.; Bianco, M.; Leandro, G.; Montalbano, L.M.; Muscatiello, N.; Monica, F.; Galeazzi, F.; et al. IBS clinical management in Italy: The AIGO survey. *Dig. Liver Dis.* **2019**, *51*, 782–789. [CrossRef]

9. Irvine, A.J.; Chey, W.D.; Ford, A.C. Screening for Celiac Disease in Irritable Bowel Syndrome: An Updated Systematic Review and Meta-analysis. *Am. J. Gastroenterol.* **2017**, *112*, 65–76. [CrossRef]
10. Bansal, A.; Sanders, D.S.; Ford, A.C. Prevalence of Irritable Bowel Syndrome–type Symptoms in Patients With Celiac Disease: A Meta-analysis. *Clin. Gastroenterol. Hepatol.* **2013**, *11*, 359–365.e1. [CrossRef]
11. Catassi, C.; Alaedini, A.; Bojarski, C.; Bonaz, B.; Bouma, G.; Carroccio, A.; Castillejo, G.; De Magistris, L.; Dieterich, W.; Di Liberto, D.; et al. The Overlapping Area of Non-Celiac Gluten Sensitivity (NCGS) and Wheat-Sensitive Irritable Bowel Syndrome (IBS): An Update. *Nutrients* **2017**, *9*, 1268. [CrossRef]
12. Dionne, J.; Ford, A.C.; Yuan, C.Y.; Chey, W.D.; Lacy, B.E.; Saito, Y.A.; Quigley, E.M.M.; Moayyedi, P. A Systematic Review and Meta-Analysis Evaluating the Efficacy of a Gluten-Free Diet and a Low FODMAPS Diet in Treating Symptoms of Irritable Bowel Syndrome. *Am. J. Gastroenterol.* **2018**, *113*, 1290–1300. [CrossRef]
13. Kelly, C.P.; Bai, J.C.; Liu, E.; Leffler, D.A. Advances in diagnosis and management of celiac disease. *Gastroenterology* **2015**, *148*, 1175–1186. [CrossRef]
14. Lebwohl, B.; Ludvigsson, J.F.; Green, P.H.R. Celiac disease and non-celiac gluten sensitivity. *BMJ* **2015**, *351*, h4347. [CrossRef] [PubMed]
15. Ford, A.C.; Chey, W.D.; Talley, N.J.; Malhotra, A.; Spiegel, B.M.; Moayyedi, P. Yield of Diagnostic Tests for Celiac Disease in Individuals With Symptoms Suggestive of Irritable Bowel Syndrome. *Arch. Intern. Med.* **2009**, *169*, 651–658. [CrossRef] [PubMed]
16. Drossman, D.A.; Camilleri, M.; Mayer, E.A.; Whitehead, W.E. AGA technical review on irritable bowel syndrome. *Gastroenterology* **2002**, *123*, 2108–2131. [CrossRef] [PubMed]
17. Spiller, R.C.; Aziz, Q.; Creed, F.; Emmanuel, A.; Houghton, L.; Hungin, P.; Jones, R.; Kumar, D.; Rubin, G.; Trudgill, N.; et al. Guidelines on the irritable bowel syndrome: Mechanisms and practical management. *Gut* **2007**, *56*, 1770–1798. [CrossRef]
18. Evidence-based position statement on the management of irritable bowel syndrome in North America. *Am. J. Gastroenterol.* **2002**, *97*, S1–S5. [CrossRef]
19. Cash, B.D.; Rubenstein, J.H.; Young, P.E.; Gentry, A.; Nojkov, B.; Lee, N.; Andrews, A.H.; Dobhan, R.; Chey, W.D. The prevalence of celiac disease among patients with nonconstipated irritable bowel syndrome is similar to controls. *Gastroenterology* **2011**, *141*, 1187–1193. [CrossRef]
20. Butterworth, J.; Iqbal, T.; Cooper, B. Coeliac disease in South Asians resident in Britain: Comparison with white Caucasian coeliac patients. *Eur. J. Gastroenterol. Hepatol.* **2005**, *17*, 541–545. [CrossRef]
21. Cranney, A.; Zarkadas, M.; Graham, I.D.; Butzner, J.D.; Rashid, M.; Warren, R.; Molloy, M.; Case, S.; Burrows, V.; Switzer, C. The Canadian Celiac Health Survey. *Dig. Dis. Sci.* **2007**, *52*, 1087–1095. [CrossRef] [PubMed]
22. Barratt, S.M.; Leeds, J.S.; Robinson, K.; Shah, P.J.; Lobo, A.J.; McAlindon, M.; Sanders, D.S. Reflux and irritable bowel syndrome are negative predictors of quality of life in coeliac disease and inflammatory bowel disease. *Eur. J. Gastroenterol. Hepatol.* **2011**, *23*, 159–165. [CrossRef] [PubMed]
23. Laurikka, P.; Salmi, T.; Collin, P.; Huhtala, H.; Mäki, M.; Kaukinen, K.; Kurppa, K. Gastrointestinal Symptoms in Celiac Disease Patients on a Long-Term Gluten-Free Diet. *Nutrients* **2016**, *8*, 429. [CrossRef] [PubMed]
24. Silvester, J.A.; Graff, L.A.; Rigaux, L.; Bernstein, C.N.; Leffler, D.A.; Kelly, C.P.; Walker, J.R.; Duerksen, D.R. Symptoms of Functional Intestinal Disorders Are Common in Patients with Celiac Disease Following Transition to a Gluten-Free Diet. *Dig. Dis. Sci.* **2017**, *62*, 2449–2454. [CrossRef]
25. Catassi, C.; Elli, L.; Bonaz, B.; Bouma, G.; Carroccio, A.; Castillejo, G.; Cellier, C.; Cristofori, F.; De Magistris, L.; Dolinšek, J.; et al. Diagnosis of Non-Celiac Gluten Sensitivity (NCGS): The Salerno Experts' Criteria. *Nutrients* **2015**, *7*, 4966–4977. [CrossRef] [PubMed]
26. Casella, G.; Villanacci, V.; Di Bella, C.; Bassotti, G.; Bold, J.; Rostami, K. Non celiac gluten sensitivity and diagnostic challenges. *Gastroenterol. Hepatol. Bed Bench* **2018**, *11*, 197–202.
27. Usai-Satta, P.; Oppia, F.; Lai, M.; Cabras, F. Motility Disorders in Celiac Disease and Non-Celiac Gluten Sensitivity: The Impact of a Gluten-Free Diet. *Nutrients* **2018**, *10*, 1705. [CrossRef]
28. Drossman, D.A. Functional Gastrointestinal Disorders: History, Pathophysiology, Clinical Features, and Rome IV. *Gastroenterology* **2016**, *150*, 1262–1279.e2. [CrossRef]
29. Böhn, L.; Störsrud, S.; Törnblom, H.; Bengtsson, U.; Simren, M. Self-Reported Food-Related Gastrointestinal Symptoms in IBS Are Common and Associated With More Severe Symptoms and Reduced Quality of Life. *Am. J. Gastroenterol.* **2013**, *108*, 634–641. [CrossRef]

30. Biesiekierski, J.R.; Peters, S.L.; Newnham, E.D.; Rosella, O.; Muir, J.G.; Gibson, P.R. No Effects of Gluten in Patients With Self-Reported Non-Celiac Gluten Sensitivity After Dietary Reduction of Fermentable, Poorly Absorbed, Short-Chain Carbohydrates. *Gastroenterology* **2013**, *145*, 320–328.e3. [CrossRef]
31. Potter, M.D.E.; Walker, M.M.; Jones, M.P.; Koloski, N.A.; Keely, S.; Talley, N.J. Wheat Intolerance and Chronic Gastrointestinal Symptoms in an Australian Population-based Study: Association Between Wheat Sensitivity, Celiac Disease and Functional Gastrointestinal Disorders. *Am. J. Gastroenterol.* **2018**, *113*, 1036–1044. [CrossRef] [PubMed]
32. Biesiekierski, J.R.; Rosella, O.; Rose, R.; Liels, K.; Barrett, J.S.; Shepherd, S.; Gibson, P.R.; Muir, J.G. Quantification of fructans, galacto-oligosaccharides and other short-chain carbohydrates in processed grains and cereals. *J. Hum. Nutr. Diet.* **2011**, *24*, 154–176. [CrossRef] [PubMed]
33. Bellini, M.; Gambaccini, D.; Bazzichi, L.; Bassotti, G.; Mumolo, M.G.; Fani, B.; Costa, F.; Ricchiuti, A.; De Bortoli, N.; Mosca, M.; et al. Bioelectrical impedance vector analysis in patients with irritable bowel syndrome on a low FODMAP diet: A pilot study. *Tech. Coloproctol.* **2017**, *21*, 451–459. [CrossRef]
34. Fritscher-Ravens, A.; Schuppan, D.; Ellrichmann, M.; Schoch, S.; Röcken, C.; Brasch, J.; Bethge, J.; Böttner, M.; Klose, J.; Milla, P.J. Confocal Endomicroscopy Shows Food-Associated Changes in the Intestinal Mucosa of Patients With Irritable Bowel Syndrome. *Gastroenterology* **2014**, *147*, 1012–1020.e4. [CrossRef] [PubMed]
35. Wu, R.L.; I Vazquez-Roque, M.; Carlson, P.; Burton, D.; Grover, M.; Camilleri, M.; Turner, J.R.; Vazquez-Roque, M. Gluten-induced symptoms in diarrhea-predominant irritable bowel syndrome are associated with increased myosin light chain kinase activity and claudin-15 expression. *Lab. Investig.* **2016**, *97*, 14–23. [CrossRef] [PubMed]
36. Elli, L.; Tomba, C.; Branchi, F.; Roncoroni, L.; Lombardo, V.; Bardella, M.T.; Ferretti, F.; Conte, D.; Valiante, F.; Fini, L.; et al. Evidence for the Presence of Non-Celiac Gluten Sensitivity in Patients with Functional Gastrointestinal Symptoms: Results from a Multicenter Randomized Double-Blind Placebo-Controlled Gluten Challenge. *Nutrients* **2016**, *8*, 84. [CrossRef] [PubMed]
37. Carroccio, A.; Mansueto, P.; Iacono, G.; Soresi, M.; D'Alcamo, A.; Cavataio, F.; Brusca, I.; Florena, A.M.; Ambrosiano, G.; Seidita, A.; et al. Non-Celiac Wheat Sensitivity Diagnosed by Double-Blind Placebo-Controlled Challenge: Exploring a New Clinical Entity. *Am. J. Gastroenterol.* **2012**, *107*, 1898–1906. [CrossRef]
38. Usai-Satta, P.; Bellini, M.; Lai, M.; Oppia, F.; Cabras, F. Therapeutic Approach for Irritable Bowel Syndrome: Old and New Strategies. *Curr. Clin. Pharmacol.* **2018**, *13*, 164–172. [CrossRef]
39. Vazquez-Roque, M.I.; Camilleri, M.; Smyrk, T.; Murray, J.A.; Marietta, E.; O'Neill, J.; Carlson, P.; Lamsam, J.; Janzow, D.; Eckert, D.; et al. A controlled trial of gluten-free diet in patients with irritable bowel syndrome-diarrhea: Effects on bowel frequency and intestinal function. *Gastroenterology* **2013**, *144*, 903–911.e3. [CrossRef]
40. Aziz, I.; Trott, N.; Briggs, R.; North, J.R.; Hadjivassiliou, M.; Sanders, D.S. Efficacy of a Gluten-Free Diet in Subjects With Irritable Bowel Syndrome-Diarrhea Unaware of Their HLA-DQ2/8 Genotype. *Clin. Gastroenterol. Hepatol.* **2016**, *14*, 696–703.e1. [CrossRef]
41. Zanwar, V.G.; Pawar, S.V.; Gambhire, P.A.; Jain, S.S.; Surude, R.G.; Shah, V.B.; Contractor, Q.Q.; Rathi, P.M. Symptomatic improvement with gluten restriction in irritable bowel syndrome: A prospective, randomized, double blinded placebo controlled trial. *Intest. Res.* **2016**, *14*, 343–350. [CrossRef] [PubMed]
42. Roncoroni, L.; Bascuñán, K.A.; Doneda, L.; Scricciolo, A.; Lombardo, V.; Branchi, F.; Ferretti, F.; Dell'Osso, B.; Montanari, V.; Bardella, M.T.; et al. A Low FODMAP Gluten-Free Diet Improves Functional Gastrointestinal Disorders and Overall Mental Health of Celiac Disease Patients: A Randomized Controlled Trial. *Nutrients* **2018**, *10*, 1023. [CrossRef] [PubMed]

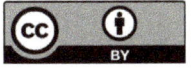

© 2020 by the authors. Licensee MDPI, Basel, Switzerland. This article is an open access article distributed under the terms and conditions of the Creative Commons Attribution (CC BY) license (http://creativecommons.org/licenses/by/4.0/).

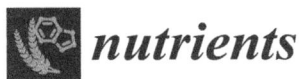

Review

Low Fermentable Oligo- Di- and Mono-Saccharides and Polyols (FODMAPs) or Gluten Free Diet: What Is Best for Irritable Bowel Syndrome?

Massimo Bellini [1], Sara Tonarelli [1,*], Maria Gloria Mumolo [1], Francesco Bronzini [1], Andrea Pancetti [1], Lorenzo Bertani [1], Francesco Costa [1], Angelo Ricchiuti [1], Nicola de Bortoli [1], Santino Marchi [1] and Alessandra Rossi [2]

- [1] Gastrointestinal Unit–Department of Translational Sciences and New Technologies in Medicine and Surgery, University of Pisa, 56124 Pisa, Italy; massimo.bellini@med.unipi.it (M.B.); g.mumolo@int.med.unipi.it (M.G.M.); bronzinifrancesco@yahoo.it (F.B.); pancio10@alice.it (A.P.); lorenzobertani@gmail.com (L.B.); fcosta@med.unipi.it (F.C.); a.ricchiuti@int.med.unipi.it (A.R.); nicola.debortoli@unipi.it (N.d.B.); santino.marchi@unipi.it (S.M.)
- [2] Clinical and Experimental Medicine–Rheumatology Unit, University of Pisa, 56100 Pisa, Italy; alessandra.rossi@unipi.it
- * Correspondence: satonarelli@gmail.com

Received: 16 September 2020; Accepted: 29 October 2020; Published: 1 November 2020

Abstract: Irritable Bowel Syndrome (IBS) is a very common functional gastrointestinal disease. Its pathogenesis is multifactorial and not yet clearly defined, and hence, its therapy mainly relies on symptomatic treatments. Changes in lifestyle and dietary behavior are usually the first step, but unfortunately, there is little high-quality scientific evidence regarding a dietary approach. This is due to the difficulty in setting up randomized double-blind controlled trials which objectively evaluate efficacy without the risk of a placebo effect. However, a Low Fermentable Oligo-, Di- and Mono-saccharides And Polyols (FODMAP) Diet (LFD) and Gluten Free Diet (GFD) are among the most frequently suggested diets. This paper aims to evaluate their possible role in IBS management. A GFD is less restrictive and easier to implement in everyday life and can be suggested for patients who clearly recognize gluten as a trigger of their symptoms. An LFD, being more restrictive and less easy to learn and to follow, needs the close supervision of a skilled nutritionist and should be reserved for patients who recognize that the trigger of their symptoms is not, or not only, gluten. Even if the evidence is of very low-quality for both diets, the LFD is the most effective among the dietary interventions suggested for treating IBS, and it is included in the most updated guidelines.

Keywords: irritable bowel disease; FODMAP; low FODMAP diet; gluten free diet; non-celiac gluten wheat sensitivity

1. Introduction

Irritable Bowel Syndrome (IBS) is one of the most common gastrointestinal disorders. Patients with IBS do not have identifiable structural or biochemical abnormalities and the diagnosis is based on the Rome IV criteria, which stress the importance of abdominal pain related to defecation and change in bowel frequency and stool consistency/form [1,2].

On the basis of the consistency/form of stools, IBS patients can be subdivided into three categories:

- IBS with predominant diarrhea (IBS-D): >25% of bowel movements with Bristol stool form types 6–7;
- IBS with predominant constipation (IBS-C): >25% of bowel movements with Bristol stool form types 1–2

- IBS with mixed bowel habits (IBS-M): >25% of bowel movements with Bristol stool form types 1 or 2 and >25% of bowel movements with Bristol stool form types 6 or 7.

If the patient cannot be categorized into one of the above three categories, he/she is defined as unclassified (IBS-U) [3].

IBS has a heterogeneous and incompletely understood pathophysiology, including altered brain-gut interactions, changes of microbiome, visceral or central hypersensitivity, abnormal gastrointestinal motility, psychosocial factors and food hypersensitivity [4]. Therefore, it is not surprising that there is no standardized and universally agreed therapy for this disorder.

However, the influence of dietary triggers on the generation of IBS symptoms has always been widely recognized [5,6]. Simren and Böhn showed that a very high percentage of IBS patients correlate their symptoms with food ingestion [7,8]. In these case studies, up to 63% and 84% of IBS patients respectively, especially women, reported food-related symptoms. Bloating and abdominal pain were the most frequently reported symptoms. Carbohydrates, fatty foods, coffee, alcohol and hot spices were the most frequently reported triggers.

The mechanisms by which food can cause symptoms in IBS patients are numerous. These include immune activation and allergy, mast cell degranulation and inflammation, luminal distension, bioactive molecules, such as peptides/amines, present in food and acting by regulating gastrointestinal motility and visceral sensitivity [9,10]. Recently, the role of Fermentable Oligo-, Di- and Mono-saccharides And Polyols (FODMAPs) have been highlighted as possible mechanisms by which food could cause symptoms in predisposed patients. These act by increasing the fluid content of the intestinal lumen due to the recall of water induced by osmotic activity, forcing water into the gastrointestinal tract and increasing the production of gas by the gut microbiota as a consequence of food fermentation [11,12].

Based on the potential role of food in symptom generation, a common therapeutic approach chosen by gastroenterologists for their IBS patients is often based on lifestyle and dietary behavior suggestions [13,14].

In recent years, many different dietary approaches have been suggested for IBS symptom improvements, such as the Low FODMAP Diet (LFD), the Gluten Free Diet (GFD), the wheat-free diet, the lactose-free diet and the NICE (National Institute for Health and Care Excellence) diet. In addition, many different do-it-yourself diets are also very frequently followed by patients, with non-scientifically motivated restrictions of one or more categories of food. These are often suggested by friends and relatives, the media and/or star system celebrities and imply a high risk of nutritional inadequacy [15].

Unfortunately, as highlighted by Dionne et al., the evidence concerning the efficacy of the different diets in IBS is often of a low quality [16].

The main limitations of clinical trials regarding the dietary therapy for IBS are:

- The difficulty in establishing an effective blinding. This is because over the years IBS patients continue or simply come to know many diets commonly suggested for IBS therapy. This makes it difficult to create a blind trial as the patients often recognize these different diets when they are suggested to the patients.
- The unclear adherence rates, except for very expensive and complex studies, such as trials that provide patients with all the food needed for the study.
- The unclear evidence about the right length of wash out period in crossover studies in order to avoid carry over effects on symptoms and also on gut microbiota.
- IBS dietary trials are rarely supported by pharmaceutical companies or investors as IBS is not seen as a profitable business.

For these reasons, IBS dietary studies are very different from one other and often include a limited number of patients. Therefore, most studies do not meet the GRADE guidelines level for high quality evidence [17].

The aim of this paper is to discuss the evidence regarding two of the most advised diets for IBS, the LFD and the GFD, in order to evaluate which of the two could be more suitable for IBS patients.

2. Gluten Free Diet

Gluten refers to a family of proteins known as prolamins (glutenin and gliadin), which are storage proteins in the starchy endosperm of many cereal grains such as wheat, barley and rye [18]. In a GFD, these cereals, and also their hybrids or derived cereals such as kamut, spelt and triticale, are not allowed. Oats are tolerated when not contaminated (however, it is necessary to check product by product). Alternatives to cereals containing gluten are rice, corn, potatoes and minor cereals or pseudocereals such as teff, millet, buckwheat, quinoa and amaranth [19]. The GFD therefore consists of a complete elimination from the diet of products containing wheat, barley and rye. This is not always simple because gluten contamination may be present in unsuspected products such as soy sauce, packet broth and malt by-products [20,21]. Table 1 reports foods that are allowed and forbidden in a GFD.

Table 1. Gluten free diet: allowed and forbidden foods.

Allowed Foods	Forbidden Foods
Corn	Wheat
Potatoes	Barley
Rice	Rye
Millet	Malt
Buckwheat	Kamut
Quinoa	Spelt
Amaranth	Triticale
Teff	Bulgur
Oats, if free from contamination	Beer
	Malt

A GFD is the only recognized therapy for Celiac Disease (CD), which is an autoimmune condition characterized by a specific serological and histological profile and triggered by gluten ingestion in genetically predisposed individuals [22]. In recent years, GFD has been suggested as a possible therapy in IBS, or at least in a subgroup of IBS patients [23] (Table 2).

Table 2. Studies on Gluten free Diet (GFD) in Irritable Bowel Syndrome (IBS).

	Patients	Methods	Evaluated Parameters	Results
Wahnschaffe et al. [24] 2001	IBS-D = 26	6 months GFD	Stool frequency IgA anti-gliadin IgA anti-tTG IEL count HLA DQ2	Improved stool frequency in patients with HLA DQ2.
Wahnschaffe et al. [25] 2007	IBS-D = 41	6 months GFD	Stool Frequency IBS symptoms questionnaire (Likert) HLA DQ2	Stool frequency and GI symptom score returned to normal values in 60% of IBS patients who were positive and in 12% who were negative for HLA DQ2.
Biesiekierski et al. [26] 2011	IBS = 34	6 weeks gluten or placebo containing bread with GFD	HLA DQ2/8 IBS symptoms questionnaire (VAS)	56% having HLA DQ2/8. 68% in the gluten group reported that symptoms were not adequately controlled compared with 40% on placebo.
Vazquez-Roque et al. [27] 2013	IBS-D = 45	4 weeks gluten containing diet or GFD	Bowel function Small bowel and colonic transit Lactulose and mannitol excretion HLA DQ2/8	The gluten containing diet increased bowel frequency in HLA DQ2/8 patients and was associated with higher intestinal permeability.

Table 2. Cont.

	Patients	Methods	Evaluated Parameters	Results
Aziz et al. [28] 2015	IBS-D = 41	6 weeks GFD	IBS-SSS HADS FIS SF-36 HLA DQ2/8	GFD reduced IBS-SSS by ≥50 points in 71%. HLA DQ2/8 positive subjects had a greater reduction in depression score and increase in vitality score.
Shahbazkhani et al. [29] 2015	IBS = 72	6 weeks GFD + 6 weeks gluten powder or placebo	IBS symptoms questionnaire (VAS)	Improvement was statistically different in the gluten containing group compared with placebo group in 25% and 83% patients, respectively.
Zanwar et al. [30] 2016	IBS = 60	4 weeks GFD + 4 weeks washout + 4 weeks DBPC rechallenge	IBS symptoms questionnaire (VAS)	Gluten group scored significantly higher in abdominal pain, bloating and tiredness and their symptoms worsened within 1 week of the rechallenge.
Barmeyer et al. [31] 2017	IBS-D/M = 35	4 months GFD	SGA IBS-SSS IBS-QoL EQ-5D HLA DQ2/8	HLA DQ2/8 was not associated with wheat sensitivity. 34% of the patients reported considerably or completely relieved symptoms on the GFD.
Paduano et al. [32] 2019	IBS = 42	4 weeks LFD + 4 weeks GFD + 4 weeks Mediterranean diet	Bristol stool scale IBS-SSS IBS-QoL IBS symptom questionnaire (VAS) SF-12	After GFD, improvement in symptoms, in particular, VAS bloating, VAS pain and IBS-SSS, with a smaller improvement in bloating compared to the low FODMAP diet, but with an adherence index of only 11%.
Pinto-Sanchez et al. [33] 2020	IBS = 50	4 weeks GFD	GI transit Birmingham IBS questionnaire Bristol Stool Scale HADS STAI-TAY PHQ-15 PGWB Anti-gliadin	After the GFD, patients with anti-gliadin reported less diarrhea. IBS symptoms improved in 75% of the patients with anti-gliadin and in 38% without the antibodies. GI transit normalized in a higher proportion of patients with anti-gliadin.

DBPC: Double-Blind Placebo-Controlled; EQ-5D: European Quality of Life-5 Dimensions; FIS: Fatigue Impact Scale; GFD: Gluten Free Diet; GI: Gastrointestinal; HADS: Hospital Anxiety and Depression Scale; HLA: Human Leukocyte Antigens; IBS: Irritable Bowel Syndrome; IBS-D: Irritable Bowel Syndrome Diarrhea; IBS-M: Irritable Bowel Syndrome Mixed; IBS-QoL: Irritable Bowel Syndrome Quality of Life; IBS-SSS: Irritable Bowel Syndrome Symptom Severity Score; IEL: Intraepithelial Lymphocytes; IgA: Immunoglobulin A; LFD: Low Fermentable Oligo-, Di- and Mono-saccharides And Polyols (FODMAP) Diet; PGWB: Psychological General Well-Being; PHQ-15: Patient Health Questionnaire; SF-12: Short Form 12; SF-36: Short Form 36; SGA: Subject's Global Assessment; STAI-TAY: State-Trait Anxiety Inventory; tTG: Tissue Transglutaminase; VAS: Visual Analogue Scale.

However, it seems important to take note of the fact that the GFD is often chosen as a "trendy diet", also by non-celiac subjects, becoming a business worth 15 million dollars in the USA only in 2016 [34,35]. One of the reasons why the GFD is so popular is because it is considered, falsely, a "miraculous" diet, improving mental and physical performances also in healthy people. On the contrary, several studies have shown that fat intake is higher than recommended and the mean intake of protein in CD patients on a GFD is lower, as well as the consumption of vegetable proteins and dietary fibers. Moreover, a higher intake of sugars and a lower intake of calcium and vitamin B12, folate and vitamin D have been reported more frequently in CD patients on a GFD than in controls [36].

Furthermore, as well as other restrictive diets, the GFD could prompt or reinforce an eating disorder [11].

3. Low FODMAP Diet

FODMAPs are a large class of small non-digestible carbohydrates containing only 1–10 sugars poorly absorbed in the small bowel. FODMAPs are common in a wide range of fruit, vegetables, cereals, milk and dairy products, legumes and sweeteners.

These molecules, found undigested in the intestinal lumen, act in different ways:

- By increasing the small bowel water content as they are osmotically active;
- By increasing the production of gas through bacterial fermentation;
- By increasing the production of bacterial metabolites such as Short-Chain Fatty Acids (SCFAs).

Within the context of visceral hypersensitivity typical of IBS patients, FODMAPs may provoke abdominal pain, bloating, flatulence and bowel habit alterations [11].

Table 3 reports allowed and forbidden foods in an LFD.

Table 3. Low FODMAP diet: Allowed and forbidden foods.

Food Categories	Allowed Foods	Forbidden Foods
Cereals	Rice, porridge, oats, quinoa, tapioca, millet, amaranth, buckwheat, gluten-free bread and cereals, potato-flour.	Bread and bakery products, biscuits, croissants, pasta, wheat flour, Kamut, barley, rye, couscous, flour, muesli.
Milk and derivates	Lactose-free milk, rice milk, oat milk, soy milk and all vegetable drinks, yogurt lactose free, soy yogurt, Greek yogurt, hard cheeses, fruit sorbets.	Cow milk, goat milk, yogurt with lactose, fresh cheeses, butter, ice cream, cream.
Vegetables	Carrot, pumpkin, Chinese cabbage, celery, lettuce, spinach, potato, tomato, zucchini, eggplant, green bean, beets, red pepper, herbs, olives, bamboo shoot, fresh herbs.	Asparagus, cauliflower, garlic, onion, shallot, mushroom, leek, chicory, fennel, artichoke, Brussel sprout, broccoli, radish, pepper, turnips, Jerusalem artichoke.
Legumes	Peas, soy products.	Beans, chickpeas, lentils, soybeans.
Fruit	Banana, blueberry, strawberry, raspberry, grape, melon, grapefruit, kiwi, orange, lemon, limes, pineapple, passion fruit.	Apple, pear, watermelon, mango, apricot, avocado, cherry, peach, plum, persimmon, lychee, fruit juices.
Dried fruits	Almonds, hazelnuts, walnuts, pine nuts.	Pistachios, cashews.
Sweeteners	White sugar, brown sugar, maple syrup.	Agave, honey, fructose, xylitol, maltitol, mannitol, sorbitol.

An LFD consists of a first phase of global elimination of all these molecules, lasting from 4 to 8 weeks, and a subsequent phase of reintegration of one category of these carbohydrates step by step. This allows the patient, who has to be followed by a skilled nutritionist, to identify the kind and the amount of foods to which he/she is sensitive, and to find adequate alternatives. This approach enables the medical practitioner to tailor the diet to the single patient. It also ensures implementation of the diet in the long term, establishing an Adapted Low FODMAP Diet (AdLFD), thus minimizing the risks of possible nutritional inadequacy [37].

The involvement of a skilled nutritionist is mandatory. This is because the reliability of information reported by patients regarding the "trigger" FODMAP-containing foods can be questionable, even in a gastroenterological setting. Indeed, Bellini et al., comparing what the patient thought before starting the LFD and the intolerance detected by the nutritionist after the reintroduction phase, found that patients' reliability in detecting the real FODMAP provoking their symptoms is generally poor or fair [38].

Although the evidence is of very low quality, an LFD had the greatest efficacy among dietary interventions suggested for treating IBS symptoms [16].

A meta-analysis by Marsh showed a significant decrease in the IBS-SSS (IBS Severity Scoring System) and an improvement in abdominal pain, bloating and IBS-QOL (IBS Quality of Life) [39].

Another meta-analysis by Schumann found that the LFD, in comparison to other diets, including the usual dietary recommendations for IBS, was effective and safe in the short term [40].

A global improvement in all parameters related to bowel habits was observed also by Bellini et al. in a group of IBS patients: the IBS-SSS global score and the scores of the single items significantly improved after the eight-week LFD [41].

However, some potential limitations and concerns of LFDs have been raised because it can

- be complex and difficult to teach and learn, because it consists of several steps and requires time, motivation and the involvement of an expert in nutritional matters;
- be potentially expensive, due to the choice of more expensive, and difficult to find alternative foods;
- reduce the normal intake of natural prebiotics, strongly modifying the gut microbiota;
- increase the risk of constipation, limiting fiber intake;
- be nutritionally inadequate;
- favor the onset of or precipitate an eating disorder behavior;
- be ineffective in the long term.

Only a few studies have assessed the long-term effects of the LFD, both in terms of efficacy and safety from a nutritional point of view [11].

In a study of our group, an eight-week LFD, monitored by a skilled nutritionist, caused no changes in energy, macronutrients or fiber intake. There were no effects on nutritional status and body composition, whereas other studies have found changes in the introduction of micro- and macronutrients during a strict LFD [41–43].

However, most of the studies that have evaluated nutritional adequacy have been based exclusively on the first phase of the LFD, while the second phase, the AdLFD, which is the diet that has to be undertaken in the long run, was rarely evaluated. Since no single food group is completely eliminated during the AdLFD, it is unlikely that patients would encounter a significant and dangerous nutritional imbalance.

In fact, O'Keeffe, evaluating the personalized diet in the long term, found no differences regarding energy and nutrient intakes between an habitual diet and an AdLFD, with higher levels of folate and vitamin A in the AdLFD [44].

Furthermore, Harvie reported that after a decrease in energy and fiber intake during the strict LFD, both energy and fiber increased to levels similar to those of the habitual diet during the AdLFD [45].

Very recently, Bellini et al., in a study involving 73 IBS patients, showed that the LFD was effective in controlling digestive symptoms both in the short and long term, and in improving quality of life, anxiety and depression, even if some problems regarding acceptability were reported and adherence decreased in the long term [38]. The diet also improved the food-related quality of life without affecting nutritional adequacy.

4. Non-Celiac Gluten/Wheat Sensitivity and IBS

A GFD is often suggested to patients with IBS-like symptoms (abdominal pain, diarrhea, bloating and flatulence). Indeed, Vazquez-Roque et al. showed that in these patients gluten caused a decrease in the expression of tight junction proteins in the colonic mucosa, causing an alteration of bowel barrier functions, especially in patients with HLA DQ8/2, the same as celiac patients [27].

In 1978, the term "Non-Celiac Gluten Sensitivity (NCGS)" was coined by Ellis and Linaker [46]. It is a clinical entity which seems often to overlap with IBS. It is characterized by gastrointestinal (GI) and extra-GI symptoms (headache, foggy mind, chronic fatigue, joint pain, tingling or numbness of the extremities, eczema) associated with gluten ingestion (occurring hours or days after the ingestion) in individuals in whom CD and wheat allergy have been excluded [47]. The diagnosis of certainty, according to the Salerno Expert consensus, is based on a close and standardized monitoring of the patient during elimination and reintroduction of gluten, in the absence of specific biomarkers [48].

This "gluten challenge" is composed of two phases (Figure 1). In the first phase patients have to maintain a gluten-containing diet for at least six weeks. After that, they start a GFD for six weeks. The second phase consists of the reintroduction of gluten (8 g of gluten per day) or placebo. For one week the patient receives the GFD and gluten or placebo, followed by a one-week washout (strict GFD) and then by the crossover with gluten or placebo for another week. In both phases the patients monitor their symptoms according to the Gastrointestinal Symptom Rating Scale (GSRS) and a Numerical Rating Scale (NRS) with a score ranging from 1 (mild) to 10 (severe). A variation in the symptom severity of at least 30% between the gluten and placebo challenge discriminates a positive from a negative result. This challenge is often performed with a single-blind approach, more suitable for clinical practice.

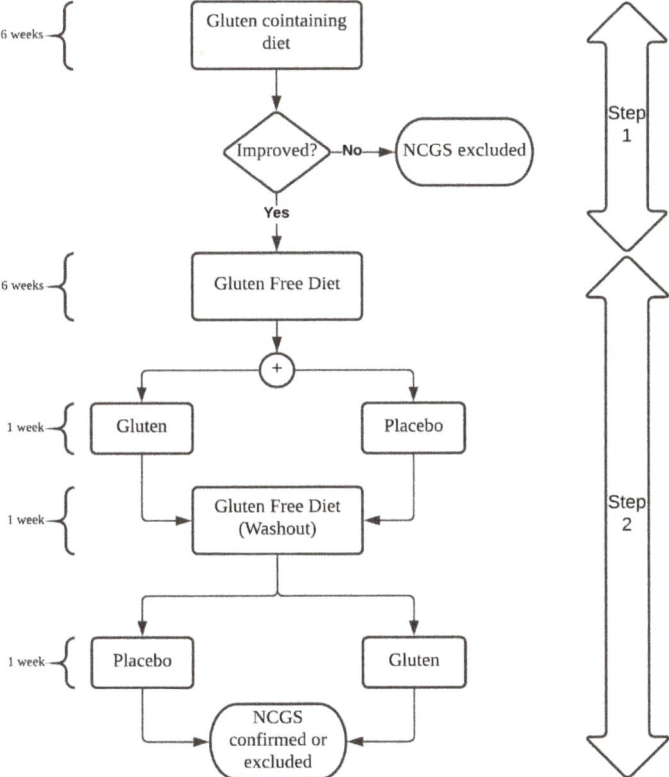

Figure 1. Gluten challenge scheme. NCGS: Non-Celiac Gluten Sensitivity.

However, the debate is still open as to whether the gluten is the culprit [30,31,48]. Indeed, also in non-gluten free food there are other molecules potentially responsible for the symptoms such as Wheat Germ Agglutinins (WGA), which induce the release of pro-inflammatory cytokines and act on the intestinal barrier, amylase trypsin inhibitors (ATIs), pest resistance molecules and activators of innate immune responses in human and murine models. Moreover, wheat also contains fructans, which are FODMAPs [49].

In 2011, Biesiekierski et al. showed that gluten caused both GI and extra-GI symptoms in non-celiac patients [26]. However, two years later, the same group reported the results of a study demonstrating that an LFD had good results in NCGS patients who had previously responded to a GFD. The symptoms then worsened with the intake of three alternative diets (low gluten, high gluten or control), with only 16% that had a worsening of symptoms in the high gluten diet. Furthermore, only a small percentage (8%) did not fail the rechallenge with gluten [50].

Some studies report that only a small percentage of patients with self-diagnosed NCGS are truly hypersensitive to gluten. In Molina-Infante's analysis, including a sample of 1312 patients, only 16% of the patients had gluten-specific symptoms, while 40% showed a nocebo response (similar or more severe symptoms in response to the placebo than with gluten) to the reintegration of gluten [51]. These results support the idea that the role of gluten is still unclear due to the high risk of placebo and nocebo effects [52].

Skodje et al. suggests that fructans are actually those most responsible for the symptoms of these patients. In a double-blind crossover challenge of 59 non-celiac subjects on a self-instituted gluten free diet the mean overall GSRS-IBS score (Gastrointestinal Symptom Rating Scale, Irritable Bowel Syndrome version) for participants consuming fructans was significantly higher than for those consuming gluten, as was the GSRS bloating sub-dimension [53]. There was no difference in GSRS-IBS scores between gluten and placebo groups. However, Volta et al. point out the limitations of this study: the authors did not use the Salerno Criteria for NCGS, but they simply enrolled self-diagnosed NCGS. In addition, some extra-GI symptoms typical of NCGS were not included in the evaluation, and data on the presence of ANCA (anti-neutrophil cytoplasmic antibodies) and anti-gliadin IgG were incomplete [54].

The results of the Skodje and Biesiekierski studies, taken together, suggest that also fructans and/or other components of wheat, and not only gluten, could be the culprits regarding the symptoms in NCGS patients. These could therefore be more precisely defined as "Non-Celiac Wheat Sensitive" (NCWS) [52].

In light of these data, NCWS patients could possibly be considered as a subset of IBS patients particularly sensitive to wheat [23].

Dieterich claims that 19 self-diagnosed NCGS patients' GSRS improved during a LFD from 13.8 ± 6.2 to 8.7 ± 5.2 ($p < 0.001$), and on a GFD (4.6 ± 4.3; $p < 0.05$), but some symptoms improved more markedly with the GFD, with both abdominal pain and alterations of bowel function responding better to the GFD [55]. This result, the LFD being more restrictive and therefore potentially more effective, is counterintuitive. However, this study did not consider the possible placebo effect that the GFD could have had in the NCGS patients. Indeed, due to the lack of blinding, the patients were able to recognize the two different diets.

It is therefore up to the clinician to understand which category each patient most likely belongs to and which diet will benefit him/her the most. This decision is fundamentally whether the patient is a NCWS patient with IBS-like symptoms responding to a GFD or is an IBS patient not sensitive to wheat or sensitive not only to wheat, for whom an LFD may be more suitable, the LFD involving a more comprehensive exclusion of potentially harmful foods. In Figure 2, a flow chart describing the management of such patients is shown.

The application in real life of a therapeutic algorithm of this kind, which includes a double-blind gluten challenge, is obviously complicated. This makes NCWS an entity of complex identification and controversial in nature, thus being closely related to the placebo/nocebo effect.

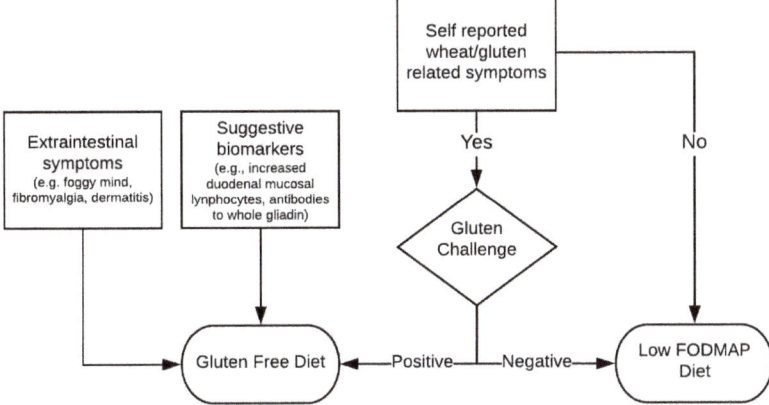

Figure 2. Algorithm for the choice between GFD and LFD in IBS.

5. Gluten Free Diet vs. Low FODMAP Diet

Therefore, what should be the most recommended diet therapy for IBS patients?

As mentioned by De Giorgio et al. and by Dionne et al., there is evidence reporting that an LFD is more effective in IBS patients than a GFD [9,16]. Recently, in a study by Paduano et al., the LFD was more effective than the GFD and a balanced diet in decreasing abdominal bloating. It was also the only regimen able to normalize the bowel function by reaching the Bristol stool form type 4 [32].

The nature of the LFD, consisting of a phase of monitored and tailored reintroduction of foods based on the tolerance/intolerance of the single patient, ensures better nutritional safety. It does not necessarily eliminate completely any category of food such as that implied by the GFD. It is however to be considered, in the choice of diet suitable for the individual patient, that in some cases, when many different foods are responsible for symptoms, even the AdLFD can be very restrictive in order to ensure a greater resolution of the symptoms.

It is consequent that even during an AdLFD in wheat-sensitive patients, it may be necessary to eliminate or greatly reduce products containing wheat. This therefore involves making extensive use of gluten-free products, which are more expensive and less nutritionally adequate than the counterparts containing gluten. This is a problem that the patients can overcome only by preparing home-made products with naturally gluten-free flours and following the suggestions of a skilled nutritionist [9,41].

Although the LFD in the first phase (the elimination of all FODMAPs) may cause an increase in spending on food, the second phase, the reintroduction phase in which a more relaxed and liberal diet is allowed, can involve reduced costs [38,44].

Evaluating the effects of both diets on the gut microbiota is difficult because studies have used different designs and methods, thus making the results not always comparable, but this is another interesting matter of discussion. A GFD seems to induce a reduction in *Bifidobacteria* and *Lactobacilli*, similarly to the LFD in the first phase [43,56,57]. Thus, as the LFD is designed to be adapted to the individual patient, with the reintroduction of a range of initially forbidden foods, it probably has a lower negative influence on gut microbiota. Harvie et al. evaluated the microbiota of patients at the end of the reintroduction of FODMAP foods and found no alteration in OTUs (Operational Taxonomic Units) after dietary intervention [45].

Finally, a GFD could be useful for those patients who report extraintestinal symptoms or have biomarkers suggesting specific symptoms (i.e., increased duodenal mucosal lymphocytes in a duodenal biopsy or serum anti-gliadin antibodies). A gluten challenge could be advisable for those reporting symptoms mainly linked to gluten ingestion, and an LFD could be directly suggested to patients without wheat/gluten related symptoms (Figure 2). This is true even if, as reported above, some evidence shows how often the perception of intolerances subjectively reported by the patients are not very reliable. Furthermore, IBS patients are not always aware of the foods really able to trigger symptoms, thus making self-diagnosed gluten intolerance somewhat unreliable [38,51].

6. Conclusions

The overlap of symptoms between NCWS and IBS, the lack of reliable markers for the diagnosis of both of them and the possibility that they could both benefit from similar types of diets generate difficulties in clearly distinguishing and characterizing this relatively new disease which deserves further studies to clarify the controversial aspects still existing. IBS patients complaining of symptoms exclusively, or mainly, linked to gluten or wheat, could benefit from a GFD as the first-line diet therapy [23]. This is because the LFD, especially in its strict phase, is a complex diet requiring close monitoring by a nutritionist expert, who is not always available. In IBS patients who report their symptoms linked to food, but not due, or not only due, to gluten/wheat ingestion, an LFD appears to be the best option. Under the careful guidance of a skilled nutritionist the LFD is nutritionally adequate and can be followed also in the long term [38]. Moreover, an LFD, with its phase of careful reintroduction of the single FODMAP categories, enables the clinician, and the patient, to have a more precise knowledge of individual sensitivity. Since the first approach to IBS patients should be based on reassurance and changes in lifestyle and dietary behavior, the LFD enables them to learn more about their own disease and about foods triggering their symptoms. However, it should be highlighted that both the GFD and LFD, as they are elimination diets, can be perceived as difficult to initiate and to continue for a lifetime by IBS patients, and consequently, their application and usefulness in daily life should be periodically and carefully monitored both by the gastroenterologist and nutritionist.

Author Contributions: Conceptualization, M.B., S.T.; review process, S.T., M.G.M., A.R. (Angelo Ricchiuti); original draft preparation, S.T., M.B., F.B.; review and editing of final manuscript, M.B., A.R. (Alessandra Rossi), S.T., L.B.; supervision M.B., F.C., A.R. (Alessandra Rossi), A.P., S.M., N.d.B. All authors have read and agreed to the published version of the manuscript.

Funding: This research received no external funding.

Acknowledgments: The authors are grateful to Chris Powell for the language revision.

Conflicts of Interest: The authors declare no conflicts of interest.

References

1. Mearin, F.; Lacy, B.E.; Chang, L.; Chey, W.D.; Lembo, A.J.; Simren, M.; Spiller, R. Bowel Disorders. *Gastroenterology* **2016**. [CrossRef]
2. Moayyedi, P.; Mearin, F.; Azpiroz, F.; Andresen, V.; Barbara, G.; Corsetti, M.; Emmanuel, A.; Hungin, A.P.S.; Layer, P.; Stanghellini, V.; et al. Irritable bowel syndrome diagnosis and management: A simplified algorithm for clinical practice. *United Eur. Gastroenterol. J.* **2017**, *5*, 773–788. [CrossRef] [PubMed]
3. Lewis, S.J.; Heaton, K.W. Stool form scale as a useful guide to intestinal transit time. *Scand J. Gastroenterol.* **1997**, *32*, 920–924. [CrossRef] [PubMed]
4. Bellini, M.; Gambaccini, D.; Stasi, C.; Urbano, M.T.; Marchi, S.; Usai-Satta, P. Irritable bowel syndrome: A disease still searching for pathogenesis, diagnosis and therapy. *World J. Gastroenterol.* **2014**, *20*, 8807–8820. [CrossRef] [PubMed]
5. Cozma-Petruţ, A.; Loghin, F.; Miere, D.; Dumitraşcu, D.L. Diet in irritable bowel syndrome: What to recommend, not what to forbid to patients! *World J. Gastroenterol.* **2017**, *23*, 3771–3783. [CrossRef] [PubMed]
6. Werlang, M.E.; Palmer, W.C.; Lacy, B.E. Irritable Bowel Syndrome and Dietary Interventions. *Gastroenterol. Hepatol. (N. Y.)* **2019**, *15*, 16–26.
7. Simrén, M.; Månsson, A.; Langkilde, A.M.; Svedlund, J.; Abrahamsson, H.; Bengtsson, U.; Björnsson, E.S. Food-related gastrointestinal symptoms in the irritable bowel syndrome. *Digestion* **2001**, *63*, 108–115. [CrossRef]

8. Böhn, L.; Störsrud, S.; Törnblom, H.; Bengtsson, U.; Simrén, M. Self-reported food-related gastrointestinal symptoms in IBS are common and associated with more severe symptoms and reduced quality of life. *Am. J. Gastroenterol.* **2013**, *108*, 634–641. [CrossRef]
9. De Giorgio, R.; Volta, U.; Gibson, P.R. Sensitivity to wheat, gluten and FODMAPs in IBS: Facts or fiction? *Gut* **2016**, *65*, 169–178. [CrossRef]
10. El-Salhy, M.; Seim, I.; Chopin, L.; Gundersen, D.; Hatlebakk, J.G.; Hausken, T. Irritable bowel syndrome: The role of gut neuroendocrine peptides. *Front. Biosci.* **2012**, *4*, 2783–2800. [CrossRef]
11. Bellini, M.; Tonarelli, S.; Nagy, A.G.; Pancetti, A.; Costa, F.; Ricchiuti, A.; de Bortoli, N.; Mosca, M.; Marchi, S.; Rossi, A. Low FODMAP Diet: Evidence, Doubts, and Hopes. *Nutrients* **2020**, *12*, 148. [CrossRef] [PubMed]
12. Gibson, P.R.; Shepherd, S.J. Personal view: Food for thought—western lifestyle and susceptibility to Crohn's disease. The FODMAP hypothesis. *Aliment. Pharmacol. Ther.* **2005**, *21*, 1399–1409. [CrossRef] [PubMed]
13. Soncini, M.; Stasi, C.; Usai Satta, P.; Milazzo, G.; Bianco, M.; Leandro, G.; Montalbano, L.M.; Muscatiello, N.; Monica, F.; Galeazzi, F.; et al. IBS clinical management in Italy: The AIGO survey. *Dig. Liver Dis.* **2019**, *51*, 782–789. [CrossRef] [PubMed]
14. Bellini, M.; Usai-Satta, P.; Bove, A.; Bocchini, R.; Galeazzi, F.; Battaglia, E.; Alduini, P.; Buscarini, E.; Bassotti, G.; ChroCoDiTE Study Group, AIGO. Chronic constipation diagnosis and treatment evaluation: The "CHRO.CO.DI.T.E." study. *BMC Gastroenterol.* **2017**, *17*, 11. [CrossRef]
15. Bellini, M.; Gambaccini, D.; Usai-Satta, P.; De Bortoli, N.; Bertani, L.; Marchi, S.; Stasi, C. Irritable bowel syndrome and chronic constipation: Fact and fiction. *World J. Gastroenterol.* **2015**, *21*, 11362–11370. [CrossRef]
16. Dionne, J.; Ford, A.C.; Yuan, Y.; Chey, W.D.; Lacy, B.E.; Saito, Y.A.; Quigley, E.M.M.; Moayyedi, P. A Systematic Review and Meta-Analysis Evaluating the Efficacy of a Gluten-Free Diet and a Low FODMAPs Diet in Treating Symptoms of Irritable Bowel Syndrome. *Am. J. Gastroenterol.* **2018**, *113*, 1290–1300. [CrossRef]
17. GRADE Working Group. Grading quality of evidence and strength of recommendations. *BMJ* **2004**, *328*, 1490. [CrossRef]
18. Niland, B.; Cash, B.D. Health Benefits and Adverse Effects of a Gluten-Free Diet in Non-Celiac Disease Patients. *Gastroenterol. Hepatol. (N. Y.)* **2018**, *14*, 82–91.
19. Saturni, L.; Ferretti, G.; Bacchetti, T. The gluten-free diet: Safety and nutritional quality. *Nutrients* **2010**, *2*, 16–34. [CrossRef]
20. Jones, A.L. The Gluten-Free Diet: Fad or Necessity? *Diabetes Spectr.* **2017**, *30*, 118–123. [CrossRef]
21. Falcomer, A.L.; Santos Araújo, L.; Farage, P.; Santos Monteiro, J.; Yoshio Nakano, E.; Puppin Zandonadi, R. Gluten contamination in food services and industry: A systematic review. *Crit. Rev. Food Sci. Nutr.* **2020**, *60*, 479–493. [CrossRef] [PubMed]
22. Caio, G.; Volta, U.; Sapone, A.; Leffler, D.A.; De Giorgio, R.; Catassi, C.; Fasano, A. Celiac disease: A comprehensive current review. *BMC Med.* **2019**, *17*, 142. [CrossRef] [PubMed]
23. Catassi, C.; Alaedini, A.; Bojarski, C.; Bonaz, B.; Bouma, G.; Carroccio, A.; Castillejo, G.; De Magistris, L.; Dieterich, W.; Di Liberto, D.; et al. The Overlapping Area of Non-Celiac Gluten Sensitivity (NCGS) and Wheat-Sensitive Irritable Bowel Syndrome (IBS): An Update. *Nutrients* **2017**, *9*, 1268. [CrossRef] [PubMed]
24. Wahnschaffe, U.; Ullrich, R.; Riecken, E.O.; Schulzke, J.D. Celiac disease-like abnormalities in a subgroup of patients with irritable bowel syndrome. *Gastroenterology* **2001**, *121*, 1329–1338. [CrossRef]
25. Wahnschaffe, U.; Schulzke, J.D.; Zeitz, M.; Ullrich, R. Predictors of clinical response to gluten-free diet in patients diagnosed with diarrhea-predominant irritable bowel syndrome. *Clin. Gastroenterol. Hepatol.* **2007**, *5*, 844–850. [CrossRef]
26. Biesiekierski, J.R.; Newnham, E.D.; Irving, P.M.; Barrett, J.S.; Haines, M.; Doecke, J.D.; Shepherd, S.J.; Muir, J.G.; Gibson, P.R. Gluten causes gastrointestinal symptoms in subjects without celiac disease: A double-blind randomized placebo-controlled trial. *Am. J. Gastroenterol.* **2011**, *106*, 508–515. [CrossRef]
27. Vazquez-Roque, M.I.; Camilleri, M.; Smyrk, T.; Murray, J.A.; Marietta, E.; O'Neill, J.; Carlson, P.; Lamsam, J.; Janzow, D.; Eckert, D.; et al. A controlled trial of gluten-free diet in patients with irritable bowel syndrome-diarrhea: Effects on bowel frequency and intestinal function. *Gastroenterology* **2013**, *144*, 903–911.e3. [CrossRef]
28. Aziz, I.; Trott, N.; Briggs, R.; North, J.R.; Hadjivassiliou, M.; Sanders, D.S. Efficacy of a Gluten-Free Diet in Subjects With Irritable Bowel Syndrome-Diarrhea Unaware of Their HLA-DQ2/8 Genotype. *Clin. Gastroenterol. Hepatol.* **2016**, *14*, 696–703.e1. [CrossRef]

29. Shahbazkhani, B.; Sadeghi, A.; Malekzadeh, R.; Khatavi, F.; Etemadi, M.; Kalantri, E.; Rostami-Nejad, M.; Rostami, K. Non-Celiac Gluten Sensitivity Has Narrowed the Spectrum of Irritable Bowel Syndrome: A Double-Blind Randomized Placebo-Controlled Trial. *Nutrients* **2015**, *7*, 4542–4554. [CrossRef]
30. Zanwar, V.G.; Pawar, S.V.; Gambhire, P.A.; Jain, S.S.; Surude, R.G.; Shah, V.B.; Contractor, Q.Q.; Rathi, P.M. Symptomatic improvement with gluten restriction in irritable bowel syndrome: A prospective, randomized, double blinded placebo controlled trial. *Intest. Res.* **2016**, *14*, 343–350. [CrossRef]
31. Barmeyer, C.; Schumann, M.; Meyer, T.; Zielinski, C.; Zuberbier, T.; Siegmund, B.; Schulzke, J.; Daum, S.; Ullrich, R. Long-term response to gluten-free diet as evidence for non-celiac wheat sensitivity in one third of patients with diarrhea-dominant and mixed-type irritable bowel syndrome. *Int. J. Colorectal. Dis.* **2017**, *32*, 29–39. [CrossRef] [PubMed]
32. Paduano, D.; Cingolani, A.; Tanda, E.; Usai, P. Effect of Three Diets (Low-FODMAP, Gluten-free and Balanced) on Irritable Bowel Syndrome Symptoms and Health-Related Quality of Life. *Nutrients* **2019**, *11*, 1566. [CrossRef] [PubMed]
33. Pinto-Sanchez, M.I.; Nardelli, A.; Borojevic, R.; de Palma, G.; Calo, N.C.; McCarville, J.; Caminero, A.; Basra, D.; Mordhorst, A.; Ignatova, E.; et al. Gluten-free Diet Reduces Symptoms, Particularly Diarrhea, in Patients with Irritable Bowel Syndrome and Anti-gliadin IgG [published online ahead of print, 2020 Aug 19]. *Clin. Gastroenterol. Hepatol.* **2020**. [CrossRef]
34. Staudacher, H.M.; Gibson, P.R. How healthy is a gluten-free diet? *Br. J. Nutr.* **2015**, *114*, 1539–1541. [CrossRef] [PubMed]
35. Rej, A.; Sanders, D.S. Gluten-Free Diet and Its 'Cousins' in Irritable Bowel Syndrome. *Nutrients* **2018**, *10*, 1727. [CrossRef]
36. Melini, V.; Melini, F. Gluten-Free Diet: Gaps and Needs for a Healthier Diet. *Nutrients* **2019**, *11*, 170. [CrossRef] [PubMed]
37. Shepard, S.; Gibson, P.; Chey, W.D. *The Complete Low-FODMAP Diet: A Revolutionary Plan for Managing IBS and Other Digestive Disorders*, 1st ed.; The Experiment LLC: New York, NY, USA, 2013.
38. Bellini, M.; Tonarelli, S.; Barracca, F.; Morganti, R.; Pancetti, A.; Bertani, L.; de Bortoli, N.; Costa, F.; Mosca, M.; Marchi, S.; et al. A Low-FODMAP Diet for Irritable Bowel Syndrome: Some Answers to the Doubts from a Long-Term Follow-Up. *Nutrients* **2020**, *12*, 2360. [CrossRef] [PubMed]
39. Marsh, A.; Eslick, E.M.; Eslick, G.D. Does a diet low in FODMAPs reduce symptoms associated with functional gastrointestinal disorders? A comprehensive systematic review and meta-analysis. *Eur. J. Nutr.* **2016**, *55*, 897–906. [CrossRef] [PubMed]
40. Schumann, D.; Klose, P.; Lauche, R.; Dobos, G.; Langhorst, J.; Cramer, H. Low fermentable, oligo-, di-, mono-saccharides and polyol diet in the treatment of irritable bowel syndrome: A systematic review and meta-analysis. *Nutrition* **2018**, *45*, 24–31. [CrossRef]
41. Bellini, M.; Gambaccini, D.; Bazzichi, L.; Bassotti, G.; Mumolo, M.G.; Fani, B.; Costa, F.; Ricchiuti, A.; De Bortoli, N.; Mosca, M.; et al. Bioelectrical impedance vector analysis in patients with irritable bowel syndrome on a low FODMAP diet: A pilot study. *Tech. Coloproctol.* **2017**, *21*, 451–459. [CrossRef]
42. Böhn, L.; Störsrud, S.; Liljebo, T.; Collin, L.; Lindfors, P.; Törnblom, H.; Simrén, M. Diet low in FODMAPs reduces symptoms of irritable bowel syndrome as well as traditional dietary advice: A randomized controlled trial. *Gastroenterology* **2015**, *149*, 1399–1407.e2. [CrossRef] [PubMed]
43. Staudacher, H.M.; Lomer, M.C.; Anderson, J.L.; Barrett, J.S.; Muir, J.G.; Irving, P.M.; Whelan, K. Fermentable carbohydrate restriction reduces luminal bifidobacteria and gastrointestinal symptoms in patients with irritable bowel syndrome. *J. Nutr.* **2012**, *142*, 1510–1518. [CrossRef] [PubMed]
44. O'Keeffe, M.; Jansen, C.; Martin, L.; Williams, M.; Seamark, L.; Staudacher, H.M.; Irving, P.M.; Whelan, K.; Lomer, M.C. Long-term impact of the low-FODMAP diet on gastrointestinal symptoms, dietary intake, patient acceptability, and healthcare utilization in irritable bowel syndrome. *Neurogastroenterol. Motil.* **2018**, *30*. [CrossRef]
45. Harvie, R.M.; Chisholm, A.W.; Bisanz, J.E.; Burton, J.P.; Herbison, P.; Schultz, K.; Schultz, M. Long-term irritable bowel syndrome symptom control with reintroduction of selected FODMAPs. *World J. Gastroenterol.* **2017**, *23*, 4632–4643. [CrossRef] [PubMed]
46. Ellis, A.; Linaker, B.D. Non-coeliac gluten sensitivity? *Lancet* **1978**, *1*, 1358–1359. [CrossRef]
47. Fasano, A.; Sapone, A.; Zevallos, V.; Schuppan, D. Nonceliac gluten sensitivity. *Gastroenterology* **2015**, *148*, 1195–1204. [CrossRef]

48. Elli, L.; Tomba, C.; Branchi, F.; Roncoroni, L.; Lombardo, V.; Bardella, M.T.; Ferretti, F.; Conte, D.; Valiante, F.; Fini, L. Evidence for the presence of non-celiac gluten sensitivity in patients with functional gastrointestinal symptoms: Results from a multicenter randomized double-blind placebo-controlled gluten challenge. *Nutrients* **2016**, *8*, 84. [CrossRef]
49. Catassi, C.; Elli, L.; Bonaz, B.; Bouma, G.; Carroccio, A.; Castillejo, G.; Cellier, C.; Cristofori, F.; de Magistris, L.; Dolinsek, J.; et al. Diagnosis of Non-Celiac Gluten Sensitivity (NCGS): The Salerno Experts' Criteria. *Nutrients* **2015**, *7*, 4966–4977. [CrossRef]
50. Biesiekierski, J.R.; Peters, S.L.; Newnham, E.D.; Rosella, O.; Muir, J.G.; Gibson, P.R. No effects of gluten in patients with self-reported non-celiac gluten sensitivity after dietary reduction of fermentable, poorly absorbed, short-chain carbohydrates. *Gastroenterology* **2013**, *145*, 320–328.e3. [CrossRef]
51. Molina-Infante, J.; Carroccio, A. Suspected Nonceliac Gluten Sensitivity Confirmed in Few Patients After Gluten Challenge in Double-Blind, Placebo-Controlled Trials. *Clin. Gastroenterol. Hepatol.* **2017**, *15*, 339–348. [CrossRef]
52. Usai-Satta, P.; Bassotti, G.; Bellini, M.; Oppia, F.; Lai, M.; Cabras, F. Irritable Bowel Syndrome and Gluten-Related Disorders. *Nutrients* **2020**, *12*, 1117. [CrossRef]
53. Skodje, G.I.; Sarna, V.K.; Minelle, I.H.; Rolfsen, K.L.; Muir, J.G.; Gibson, P.R.; Veierød, M.B.; Henriksen, C.; Lundin, K.E.A. Fructan, Rather Than Gluten, Induces Symptoms in Patients With Self-Reported Non-Celiac Gluten Sensitivity. *Gastroenterology* **2018**, *154*, 529–539.e2. [CrossRef]
54. Volta, U.; Caio, G.; De Giorgio, R. More Than One Culprit for Nonceliac Gluten/Wheat Sensitivity. *Gastroenterology* **2018**, *155*, 227. [CrossRef]
55. Dieterich, W.; Schuppan, D.; Schink, M.; Schwappacher, R.; Wirtz, S.; Agaimy, A.; Neurath, M.F.; Zopf, Y. Influence of low FODMAP and gluten-free diets on disease activity and intestinal microbiota in patients with non-celiac gluten sensitivity. *Clin. Nutr.* **2019**, *38*, 697–707. [CrossRef]
56. McIntosh, K.; Reed, D.E.; Schneider, T.; Dang, F.; Keshteli, A.H.; De Palma, G.; Madsen, K.; Bercik, P.; Vanner, S. FODMAPs alter symptoms and the metabolome of patients with IBS: A randomised controlled trial. *Gut* **2017**, *66*, 1241–1251. [CrossRef]
57. Nistal, E.; Caminero, A.; Herrán, A.R.; Arias, L.; Vivas, S.; de Morales, J.M.; Calleja, S.; de Miera, L.E.; Arroyo, P.; Casqueiro, J. Differences of small intestinal bacteria populations in adults and children with/without celiac disease: Effect of age, gluten diet, and disease. *Inflamm. Bowel Dis.* **2012**, *18*, 649–656. [CrossRef] [PubMed]

Publisher's Note: MDPI stays neutral with regard to jurisdictional claims in published maps and institutional affiliations.

© 2020 by the authors. Licensee MDPI, Basel, Switzerland. This article is an open access article distributed under the terms and conditions of the Creative Commons Attribution (CC BY) license (http://creativecommons.org/licenses/by/4.0/).

MDPI
St. Alban-Anlage 66
4052 Basel
Switzerland
Tel. +41 61 683 77 34
Fax +41 61 302 89 18
www.mdpi.com

Nutrients Editorial Office
E-mail: nutrients@mdpi.com
www.mdpi.com/journal/nutrients

www.ingramcontent.com/pod-product-compliance
Lightning Source LLC
LaVergne TN
LVHW070547100526
838202LV00012B/403